A Short Textbook
Ear Nose and Throat

R. Pracy

F.R.C.S.,
Consultant
Oto-rhino-laryngologist,
Hospital for Sick
Children, and The
Royal National Throat,
Nose and Ear Hospital,
London

J. Siegler

F.R.C.S., D.L.O.,
Consultant
Oto-rhino-laryngologist
Liverpool Health
Authority (Teaching)

P. M. Stell

Ch.M., F.R.C.S.,
Professor of
Oto-rhino-laryngology,
University of Liverpool

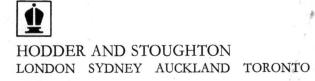

HODDER AND STOUGHTON
LONDON   SYDNEY   AUCKLAND   TORONTO

Editor's Foreword

The familiar green paper-backs of the Short Textbook Series have become an established feature of the modern medical library and few students do not have at least one of the volumes on their shelves.

The Short Textbook of Surgery does not include a section on otorhinolaryngology and the gap has now been filled by this book. The authors have tackled a difficult task in an original yet simple manner. What to most appears at first a complicated subject, has been reduced to its most elementary by the skilful use of line illustrations and a brief supporting text. One page of really good diagrams is worth five pages of text and so here we have multum in parvo.

There is no doubt that this, the latest addition to the green-backs will be a very welcome and equally popular publication.

SELWYN TAYLOR

Preface

Although there are already several textbooks of Ear Nose and Throat Surgery for the undergraduate, all are expensive and most are more comprehensive than the average undergraduate probably needs.

We feel, therefore, that there is a need for a textbook which can be easily read, and we have tried to produce a short inexpensive book which explains the diseases of the ears, nose and throat which are commonly seen by a general practitioner and which the undergraduate should therefore understand.

We should like to express our thanks to F. Ronald Edwards, M.D., Ch.M., F.R.C.S., for his contribution to the chapter on Dysphagia, to Mr. J. H. Rogers, F.R.C.S., for his help with the proofs and the preparation of the Index, and to Dr. R. A. Yorston of Dundee for the preparation of the illustrations.

R. PRACY, J. SIEGLER, P. M. STELL

Contents

Chapter One
Symptoms and signs of ear diseases

SYMPTOMS OF EAR DISEASE
The main symptoms of ear disease are earache, deafness, discharge, vertigo and tinnitus.

Earache
Earache is usually due to otitis media, a boil or impacted wax. Pain may be referred to the ear from disease elsewhere in the upper respiratory tract, so that a carcinoma of the posterior third of tongue, a carcinoma of tonsil or a carious molar tooth should be borne in mind when the ear looks normal on examination. Figure 1 shows the causes of earache.

Deafness
An elderly adult often refuses to admit to being deaf, and his friends have to persuade him to seek advice. Listening to people becomes difficult because discrimination of speech is lost and everything sounds muffled.

A young adult needs good hearing for his work, and therefore comes willingly and early for advice.

A child may be found to be deaf during a routine audiometric test at school, or his teacher may find that he is inattentive or backward in class work. His parents may complain that he does not obey them, or that he increases the sound in order to hear the television.

Discharge
Discharge from an ear may be watery, purulent, mucopurulent, foul or blood-stained.

A watery discharge is usually due to diffuse external otitis and often causes crusting at the orifice.

A purulent discharge comes from a boil in the canal.

A mucopurulent discharge comes from the middle ear during acute or benign chronic suppurative otitis media. It is pale yellow, tenacious and *odourless*.

A foul-smelling discharge is evidence of attic cholesteatoma or marginal granulations.

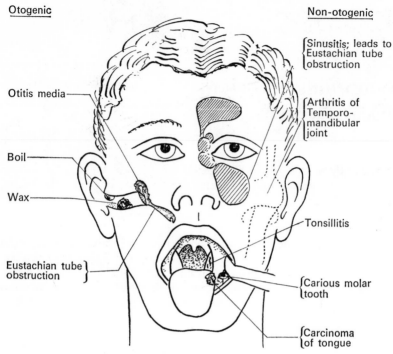

Otogenic

Non-otogenic

Sinusitis; leads to Eustachian tube obstruction

Otitis media

Arthritis of Temporo-mandibular joint

Boil

Wax

Eustachian tube obstruction

Tonsillitis

Carious molar tooth

Carcinoma of tongue

Fig. 1 Causes of earache.

A blood-stained discharge is due to an aural polyp or acute otitis media, with bleeding into the middle ear. A carcinoma of the ear may cause bleeding, but this is uncommon.

Tinnitus (noises in the ear)
Tinnitus is complained of very often, especially in old people suffering from presbycusis. It causes a lot of distress, especially at night when the patient is trying to sleep. Many patients have no abnormality in their ears or upper respiratory tract, but it may occur in otosclerosis and in chronic otitis media.

Vertigo
Vertigo is a sensation of abnormal movement of the surroundings in relation to the patient, or of the patient in relation to his surroundings. It will be described in another chapter.

CLINICAL EXAMINATION
External inspection
Much may be learned by looking at the ear with a good light. The orifice may show crusting or weeping due to external otitis; it may be

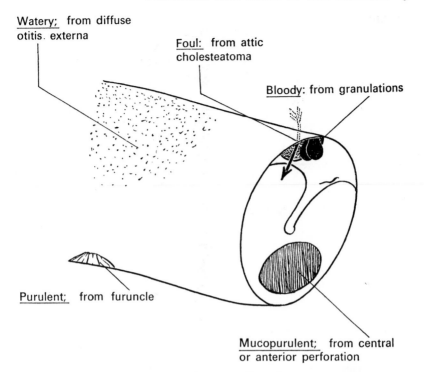

Watery; from diffuse otitis externa

Foul: from attic cholesteatoma

Bloody: from granulations

Purulent; from furuncle

Mucopurulent; from central or anterior perforation

Fig. 2 Types and sources of otorrhoea.

enlarged by a mastoid operation, or swollen and narrowed by a boil. The pinna should always be folded forwards to look for the scar of a previous mastoid operation. When the patient is suffering from acute earache look for swelling or tenderness over the mastoid process.

Internal examination
To get a clear view of the drum, the pinna and cartilaginous canal must be pulled upwards and backwards. This will create a straight line from the orifice to the drum. In a very young baby the pinna should be pulled downwards and forwards.

Children often resent having their ears examined despite gentle handling. It may be difficult to examine an ear because:

1 The canal is full of wax.
2 The canal is too narrow.
3 The speculum is too large and will not enter the bony canal. The skin bulges into the end of the speculum and obstructs the view.

There are two sets of instruments generally used for examination of an ear. The electric auriscope gives an excellent enlarged view of the drum and can be used without special training. Both hands are needed, making it impossible to remove wax.

A head mirror, focusing lamp and a Siegel's aural speculum are used in otological clinics. They are difficult to use at first, but the student can handle them with ease after a little guidance. The main advantages are:

1 The canal and drum can be seen without a speculum, if the canal is wide enough.
2 The otologist has a free hand to clean the canal even if a speculum is needed.

The disadvantages are that much equipment is needed for a simple examination. It is also necessary to magnify the drum by attaching a lens to the speculum. Failure to do this may cause a perforation to be missed.

Appearance of a normal tympanic membrane

The major part of the tympanic membrane, the pars tensa, is a pale grey tense thin membrane, attached to the tympanic ring. The part of the tympanic membrane covering the attic region, the pars flaccida, is loose and much thicker. In the centre of the tympanic membrane, the white handle of the malleus stands out in contrast to the rest of the tympanic membrane. The short, lateral process of the malleus projects laterally from the upper end of the handle and thickenings in the tympanic membrane known as the anterior and posterior malleolar folds pass forwards and backwards from the lateral process. A triangular-shaped cone of light passes downwards and forwards from the umbo at the lower end of the handle of the malleus.

Examination of ear with an operating microscope

In modern otological clinics a microscope is essential to inspect all quadrants of the drum adequately. Pus and debris may be aspirated and disease in the attic, margin or centre of the tympanic membrane confirmed.

Mobility of drum

Healed perforations and scars are seen when the tympanic membrane is moved by applying positive and negative pressure. To do this the speculum must fit tightly in the canal. A magnifying lens with side attachment for a rubber suction bulb is fitted into the opening; squeezing the bulb then causes the tympanic membrane to move.

Examination of the upper respiratory tract is a vital step in the investigation of ear symptoms. In a child, the adenoidal pad and sinusitis can cause recurrent otitis media; in an adult, carcinoma of the post-nasal space may cause conductive deafness.

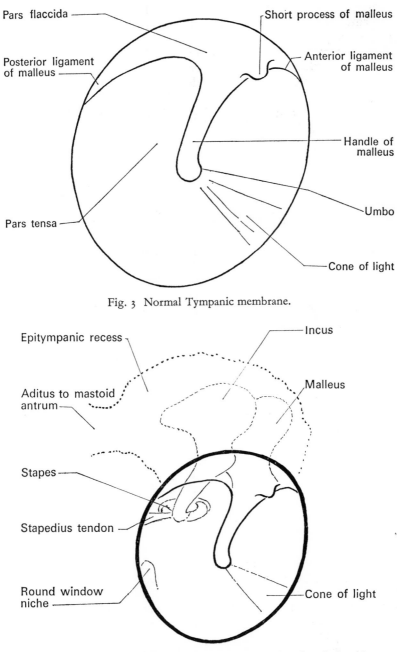

Fig. 3 Normal Tympanic membrane.

Fig. 4 Diagram of Rt. Tympanic membrane showing the relationship of the auditory ossicles.

HEARING TESTS

Measuring and localizing deafness

1 Testing a patient's response to whispered voice is rough indication of deafness. The opposite ear must be masked by rubbing a piece of paper over it. The patient looks away from the examiner and repeats a series of numbers or simple words such as 'cat', 'dog' or 'house', which are whispered into the ear to be tested. The farthest distance away from the ear that the words can just be heard is recorded. A quiet room is essential for concentration and exclusion of other sounds. The normal ear hears a whisper at five feet (1·5 metres).

2 Testing response to *conversational* voice is carried out in the same way, this time using ordinary speaking voice which a normal ear should hear at thirty feet (9 metres).

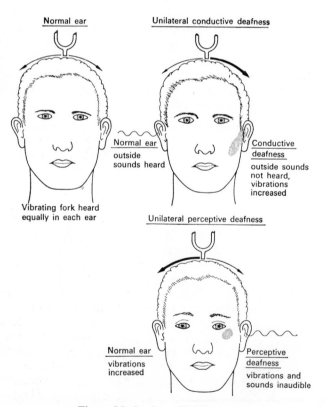

Fig. 5 Mechanism of Weber test.

Weber test

The base of a vibrating fork is placed on the centre of the forehead. The sound waves pass across the skull towards both ears and are heard equally if the hearing is normal. Conductive deafness in one ear causes the vibrations to be heard louder on that side (see Fig. 5). If there is a unilateral perceptive deafness the sound is heard better on the normal side.

Mechanism

Bone conduction has two components: (1) direct, to cochlea; and (2) indirect, to middle ear. Part of the indirect component is directed to the cochlea, but most of it is dissipated to the outer ear. In the inner ear disease, the cochlear part of the indirect component is too weak to stimulate the cochlea, and so the sound appears louder in the good ear. In middle ear disease, the middle ear part of the indirect component cannot dissipate into the outer ear, and is therefore added to the cochlear component. The sound therefore appears louder in the affected ear.

Rinne's test

This test shows whether the deafness is conductive or perceptive. The prongs of a vibrating tuning fork are held beside the ear and the base then placed on the mastoid process. The patient is asked to compare the intensity of sound heard at the two positions—a patient with conductive deafness hears the sound better when the fork is placed over the mastoid process than when placed beside the ear. In perceptive deafness the findings are reversed.

Absolute bone conduction (A.B.C.)

The length of time during which the patient hears the vibrations when the base of a tuning fork is placed on the mastoid process is compared to the time heard by the observer. In a conductive deafness, the length of time the patient hears the fork is prolonged, in a perceptive deafness it is shortened.

Audiometry

An audiometer is an electronic instrument producing pure tones by means of an oscillator. The intensity of the notes produced can be altered and is measured in decibels. A normal conversation is heard over the spectrum of 500, 2000, 4000 cycles/second.

It is necessary to take audiograms in a silent room and every otological clinic should be equipped with one. Outside hospital a quiet room away from traffic may suffice. Earphones worn by the patient are connected to the audiometer. The patient listens until the sound first appears and then until it just disappears. The measurement of these two thresholds is the hearing loss for that frequency. It is estimated first for air conduction, and then for bone conduction, at each of the above frequencies. For examples of audiograms see Appendix, p. 153.

Chapter Two
Deafness in the young child

INTRODUCTION

This chapter deals with the effects of permanent deafness in the young child. Temporary or variable deafness in children will be dealt with elsewhere (*vide* Chapter Four).

The incidence of such deafness is 1 : 10 000 population. Usually the mother who brings her child for advice because of deafness does not complain that he cannot hear but rather that he does not SPEAK. Before discussing, therefore, the methods of investigation of such a patient we must describe how the child acquires speech and language.

NORMAL DEVELOPMENT OF SPEECH AND HEARING

The new-born baby responds to loud sounds with a startle or Moro reflex. He cannot localise sounds. Over the first four months of life he becomes accustomed to the noises in the immediate environment and towards the end of this period begins to associate certain noises with certain objects or persons. Thus he may turn his head towards the sound of a spoon 'chinked' against the feeding cup. He may turn the head to the sound of a rattle. He will only turn, however, to sounds made at 'ear level'; he cannot locate sounds made above the head. Between six and eight months the normal child begins to experiment in the use of the voice. He phonates, making such sounds as Ma ma ma and Da da da and ba ba ba, repeating them with pleasure. Not only does he experiment in consonant/vowel associations but also experiments in varying pitch, so that he can frequently be heard 'accelerating' up the scale. It is physiological for the child to make these sounds spontaneously but he will only continue to do so if he can HEAR the sounds so made. In other words, the sound is 'fed back' to the infant through his own skeleton to the hearing organ. This is how man modulates the sounds of speech.

At about twelve months of age the average child says his first word. Gradually over the next six months he adds another five words. At two years of age he has twenty-four words and at three years of age he has three hundred words. Between three years and five and a half years

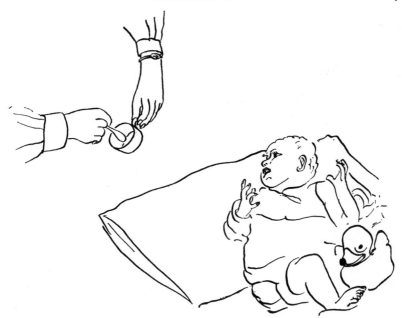

Fig. 6 Response to meaningful sound.

LANGUAGE is acquired. The average child's response to sound is sum-
marised in Table 1 as:

TABLE I

at birth	startle response to loud sound
at four months	will turn head to meaningful sounds at the ear level
at six to eight months	babbles Ma ma ma, etc.
at one year	one word
at eighteen months	six words
at two years	twenty-four words
at three years	three hundred words
between three and five and a half years	acquires language

It is fundamental to realise that he will only pass these auditory landmarks if he is of normal intelligence. The figures in Table 1 are the
average, therefore, for a child with an intelligence quotient of 100.

The dilemma which confronts the doctor faced with the problem
child who does not speak is—is the child deaf or is the child backward
or has the child an aphasia?

Unfortunately a child who is backward may not pass the ordinary auditory milestones at the usual age and his environment may be so small that he does not respond to quiet sounds at a distance.

We have, therefore, now to tabulate some of the physical milestones through which the child should pass if physical development is normal.

TABLE 2

focuses eyes	six weeks
raises head	three to four months
sits up unaided	six to eight months
stands	ten to twelve months
walks	twelve to fourteen months
feeds himself	twelve to eighteen months
is clean and dry	two to three years

AETIOLOGY OF CONGENITAL DEAFNESS

The vast majority of cases of congenital deafness are of the nerve or perceptive type. Some types run in families (e.g. Waardenburg's Syndrome—different-coloured irises, a white streak in the hair and perceptive deafness). Some result from the exposure of the mother to ototoxic agents during the 'ear-forming' stage of her pregnancy (six to twelve weeks). This may be seen in the child of the mother who has rubella at this time. Occasionally deafness is due to maternal syphilis. Many cases result from perinatal hypoxia in the infant. This may be due to such factors as Rhesus incompatibility or perinatal asphyxia, but in either event the cause of the deafness is lack of oxygenation and death of the nerve cells. When all of these infants have been allotted to their various groups there will remain a large number for whom there is no clear indication as to the causative factor. The largest group of deaf children is that group in which no cause can be found.

ASSESSMENT OF DEAFNESS

From what has been said already it is obvious that the task of the doctor in assessing possible deafness in the young child is complex. What he has to try to demonstrate is that only those skills subserved by hearing are lacking in the child's development. This may be extremely difficult and it requires the co-operation of many different disciplines. A typical 'assessment team' consists of a paediatrician, an educational psychologist, a teacher of the deaf, a school medical officer and an otologist. No one of these people is more important than another. Frequently a small child is overawed by so many people, and so while the response to sound is being observed only one of the team stays in the room with the child. The other members remain outside in an observation chamber with a two-way communication channel.

Before the response to sound is ascertained, the medical members of the team question the mother. The information they require is:

1 How was the deafness first suspected? What is the response to sound?

2 At what age have the other physical developmental landmarks been passed? How do these compare with siblings?

3 Is there a family history of deafness?

4 Was the mother ill during the second/third month of pregnancy? Did she receive drugs at that time? Is the mother Rhesus positive or negative?

5 Did the pregnancy proceed to full term? Was there possible toxaemia?

6 Was the birth normal? Did the child breathe at once? Was there any perinatal hypoxia?

7 Has the child had any severe illness since birth?

Once the answers to these questions have been collated the patient is examined. Note is taken of his general physical state and of the stage of muscle control and stability. The ears, nose and throat are examined to exclude possible causes of conductive deafness. The eyes, heart and lungs are examined for possible defects.

While the mother is questioned, the child will have settled down in the assessment room and will be playing with the toys there.

The next stage in the assessment is to 'spray' the child with sound. Variable pitches and variable intensities of sound are fed in from all angles and the response noted by each observer. The only POSITIVE response is the one which satisfies every member of the team.

For the child up to nine months of age the test sounds will include

    cup and spoon chinked together
    high- and low-pitch rattles
    crumpling paper
    ringing of bells
    playing of a musical box
    calling his name
    hissing

All these sounds must be made at 'ear level' in order to check that each ear is turned to the sound stimulus. Until nine months of age the child is unable to locate sounds which are not at ear level.

After nine months a variety of sounds may be used, including speech and music fed through an amplifier system, drums, rattles and xylophones.

As the child grows older it can be engaged in a 'go game'. The basis of this 'game' is that as soon as the child hears a sound it performs some simple act such as taking a peg from a peg-board and putting it into a box or removing a doll from a toy bus. The sound stimulus can be varied in pitch and intensity, and the degree of loudness measured with a sound-level meter. In this way it may be possible to draw a simple audiogram.

It is not usually possible to do a formal 'Pure Tone Audiogram' using head-phones and an audiometer until the child is four years old or more. Although it is obviously important for the patient that deafness should be diagnosed at any age, it is too late to wait until four years of age before getting an accurate picture of the degree of hearing loss. It is too late because four years of that period of life in which the child develops speech as a response to sound have passed. There are only eighteen months left for the child to acquire not only speech but also language, and even with the most intelligent child and the most understanding teacher this is just not enough time. After five and a half the child will begin to lose the ability to develop language. From what has been said already it will be apparent that the diagnosis of deafness in a child may be difficult, and indeed it may not be possible on the first attendance. If this is so, then it is necessary for mother and child to attend repeatedly, until the assessors are satisfied that the child is or is not deaf.

TREATMENT

Where deafness is diagnosed it is frequently severe, and nerve deafness, with which we are concerned in this chapter, usually affects the higher sounds to a greater extent than the lower frequencies. That is to say that the child is more likely to hear vowel sounds than consonants. As Fig. 7 shows, consonants are of high pitch and low intensity. Vowel sounds are of low pitch and high intensity.

If, therefore, he is to be fitted with a hearing aid it should boost the high frequency sounds to a greater extent than the low frequencies.

Once deafness is diagnosed, the child is fitted with a hearing aid. Plastic inserts should be made for each ear, and probably it is of benefit if the child has two separate hearing aids, one for each ear in order to provide 'stereophonic sound'. However, this has never been proved, and most deaf children do very well with a simple hearing aid fitted with a 'Y' lead to two ear receivers. However, the simple provision of a hearing aid with a 'Y' lead does not compensate completely for the handicap of deafness and it is most important that the education of the MOTHER and CHILD in the use of the aid should begin at once. Thus it is that most local authorities provide mother and child training and pre-school training facilities for the deaf child. In the former the mother and child attend once or twice weekly for individual tuition with a teacher of the deaf. In the latter the child is admitted to a nursery class and begins his education with other children. This usually occurs at the age of two to two and a half years.

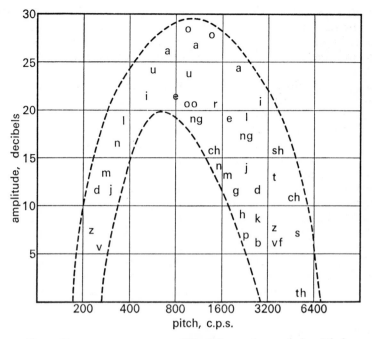

Fig. 7 Frequency components of English speech sounds (modified from Watkyn-Thomas, Fig. 262, p. 504).

If the child has a deafness of only moderate severity and if this is detected early and auditory training started promptly, then it may be possible for him to be educated in an ordinary school with hearing children. This would certainly be the ideal place for him. However, many children are severely deaf and for them formal education can be provided only in a specially treated classroom fitted with speech trainers. The teachers must be specially trained to teach deaf children. The classes must be small (usually about eight children in a class). The education is always a slow process and the deaf child is required by law to stay at school until after his sixteenth birthday.

In the past fifty years great progress has been made in the education of the deaf child, and if similar progress is made in the next fifty years we may look forward to the virtual disappearance of this serious social handicap.

Chapter Three
Diseases of the external ear

ANATOMICAL SUMMARY

The external ear consists of the pinna and the external auditory canal. The pinna and the outer one-third of the external canal are supported by elastic cartilage to which the skin is densely adherent. In the outer cartilaginous part of the canal the skin has subcutaneous tisssue, hairs and ceruminous glands. The skin lining the inner bony part of the canal is very thin and is attached to the periosteum; it has neither hairs nor glands. For these anatomical reasons, wax and boils form in the outer part of the canal and bony atresia occurs in the inner third.

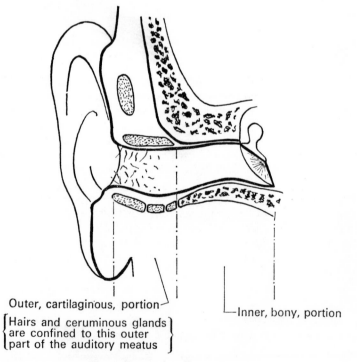

Outer, cartilaginous, portion
{ Hairs and ceruminous glands are confined to this outer part of the auditory meatus }
Inner, bony, portion

Fig. 8 External auditory meatus.

WAX

Wax is the normal secretion of the ceruminous glands lining the carti-laginous canal. The quantity and consistency vary considerably.
Clinical picture. Wax can cause deafness, earache, discharge and vertigo, despite being a normal secretion. The quantity secreted and the con-sistency vary so that many people need syringing of their ears at regular intervals.
Soft wax is removed easily with a probe covered with cotton wool.
Hard wax must be softened before being syringed. The ear is filled with 10 % solution of soap in water. The drops are massaged into the wax and left there for twenty minutes. The ear is then syringed and examined to confirm total removal of wax without damage to the drum, although the meatus and drum will be red.
Very hard wax will need to be softened for five days before syringing. The patient uses the drops himself as described.
Removal of wax under a general anaesthetic may be necessary when syring-ing is unsuccessful. Syringing an ear that is filled with hard impacted wax causes severe pain. It may then be necessary to remove the wax under a general anaesthetic. This is frequently necessary when hard wax is covered by a layer of keratin.

DISEASES

Foreign bodies

A child may put a foreign body into its ear while playing. Beads, parts of plastic toys or the ends of pencils are often found. They do not cause symptoms.

Treatment

Syringing will remove most foreign bodies unless they are impacted in the deep canal. In this case the patient should be referred to an otolo-gist, who will remove the foreign body under a general anaesthetic. There is a serious risk of perforation of the drum when an attempt is made to remove the foreign body in the casualty room. An organic foreign body, such as a pea, should not be syringed as water will make it swell and it should be removed by an otologist.

Trauma

The pinna may be injured during boxing or an assault; a haematoma collects beneath the skin. Several aspirations are necessary to prevent a cauliflower ear deformity as a result of the blood clot becoming organised.
The lobe may be badly lacerated and remain attached to the pinna by a narrow bridge of skin. It should be sutured to the pinna and will probably heal satisfactorily. The patient should be given a course of antibiotics to prevent perichondritis.

The canal may be injured while removing wax with a hair grip or during syringing. A piece of cotton wool kept at the orifice will prevent the laceration becoming infected. The patient is given a course of Penicillin for prophylaxis.

Infections

Localised external otitis (*syn. boil*) is due to infection of a hair follicle in the cartilaginous external canal by *Staphylococcus aureus*.

This causes severe earache, made worse by moving or touching the pinna. The orifice is red and swollen. Sometimes the swelling spreads to the tissues behind the ear and resembles acute mastoiditis. Severe pain is caused by inserting an ear speculum.

Treatment
Pain must be relieved by soluble Aspirin or Paracetamol given every four hours. Wicks soaked in Glycerine and Mag. Sulph. Paste (B.P.) are gently placed in the canal each day. These help to draw the infection out of the hair follicle. Intramuscular Penicillin 500 000 units should also be given every six hours.

Should the patient suffer from recurrent boils in the ears, a nasal swab should be taken to exclude organisms, usually staphylococci, being carried in the nasal vestibule. An antiseptic ointment should be prescribed for carriers. The urine must be examined to exclude glycosuria.

Diffuse external otitis may involve one or both ears.
Unilateral is often secondary to an underlying otitis media.
Bilateral may be due to bacterial or fungal infection, reaction of the skin to a chemical irritant or part of a generalised skin disorder. It is often associated with emotional upsets.
Bacterial external otitis usually follows scratching the skin while removing wax with a kirby grip. Further irritation follows and the patient is compelled to scratch his ear again. Pus collects in the canal and the skin becomes red and swollen.
Fungal external otitis following swimming in the tropics is due to infection with the fungus *Aspergillus niger*. The canal becomes filled with white debris covered with black spots, comparable to wet blotting paper.
Chemical irritants such as hair dyes, hair lacquers and local antibiotics sensitise the skin and cause a local dermatitis.

Clinical picture
The patient complains of severe irritation in both ears; he feels compelled to scratch his ears, especially while in bed. His ears discharge and he is often deaf. The canals are full of debris with inflammation of the meatal skin. The deafness is relieved after the canals have been cleaned.

Treatment
Careful aural toilet followed by a dressing soaked in 1% Mercuro-chrome will help most patients. The aural toilet should be repeated each day until the infection has resolved. *Aspergillus niger* requires dressings soaked in 2% Salicylic Acid in Spirit or Nystatin. Water should be prevented from entering the ear for one month.

Acute perichondritis is an unusual ear infection. The cartilage may become infected after a radical mastoid operation for chronic otitis media. The cartilage has been exposed while the orifice is being enlarged and subsequently becomes infected.

Clinical picture
The patient suffers severe pain in the pinna, which becomes red, swollen and tender. The lobule is not involved.

Treatment
A course of Tetracycline 250 mg six-hourly should be started immediately and continued for ten days. The pinna should be examined daily for abscess formation, which requires incision and drainage. Unfortunately, many patients are left with an ear deformed by scar tissue.

Tumours of the external ear

Pinna
Benign
A papilloma usually arises at the orifice of the canal. It is a simple wart and is treated by removal under a local anaesthetic.

Malignant
(a) *Carcinoma* may follow on a rodent ulcer or an area of keratosis. A squamous carcinoma is the commonest malignant tumour arising from the pinna, although a basal cell carcinoma is much more common over the rest of the face. It is usually a papilliferous mass with central ulceration which bleeds when touched. The early carcinoma does not cause pain. Later, after invasion of the cartilage, the patient suffers intense pain.
(b) *Rodent ulcer* occurs among patients who have worked for many years in strong sunlight. The ulcer shows the typical rolled edge with crusting in the centre.

Treatment
An early superficial carcinoma responds to radiotherapy.
A more extensive tumour with the invasion of the cartilage requires removal of part or the whole of the pinna.

Canal

Benign

Osteomata grow in the deep bony canal. They are usually sessile, made of compact bone and are often seen in patients who have swum often. There are frequently two or three in each ear.

Clinical picture

The patient may be unaware of them if small. The osteomata may grow and cause retention of wax on the surface of the drum. External otitis may follow and the osteomata should be removed.

Malignant

Carcinoma may arise in the external canal or invade the canal from the middle ear. The patient suffers intense earache. The ear discharges pus and blood. Sometimes he develops a facial nerve paralysis. A radical mastoid operation is necessary, followed by a course of radio-therapy.

Chapter Four
Acute diseases of the middle ear cleft

There are two common acute diseases of the middle ear cleft: secretory otitis media and acute suppurative otitis media. Both are common diseases of childhood, and in both obstruction of the Eustachian tube is an important factor.

SECRETORY OTITIS MEDIA
Secretory otitis media is a common cause of deafness in childhood.

Pathology
Obstruction of the Eustachian tubes, due to a cold, enlarged adenoid or infected sinuses, prevents air from entering the middle ear as normally happens when the patient swallows. Partial reabsorption of the air remaining in the middle ear follows, causing a vacuum. As a result of this vacuum the tympanic membrane becomes indrawn and there is an effusion into the middle ear.

Clinical features
This is a common cause of deafness in childhood and there are usually no other symptoms; although there is no pain the patient may complain of dullness of the ear. The ear never discharges. There are also the symptoms of the underlying disease such as enlarged adenoid, chronic sinusitis, etc.

Examination of the tympanic membrane shows it to be indrawn and it may appear golden in colour because of the effusion in the middle ear. If there is intermittent air entering into the ear, a fluid level may be seen.

Tuning fork tests and audiometry show the deafness to be conductive in type. (See Appendix 1.)

The nose and throat should be examined to determine the cause of the obstruction of the Eustachian tube.

The disease is less common in adults and if unilateral a carcinoma of the nasopharynx should be suspected.

Treatment
The underlying cause should be treated as indicated. This will usually mean an antrum wash-out and removal of the adenoids.

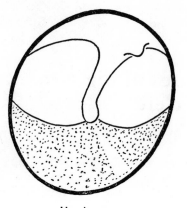

Head erect

Fig. 9 Fluid in Tympanic cavity.

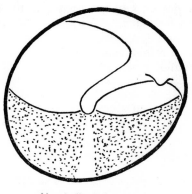

Head tilted forward

Fig. 10 Fluid in Tympanic cavity.

The fluid in the middle ear is removed by a myringotomy and suction. The disease affects children at the age when lymphoid hyperplasia is maximal, that is from five to seven years. If it recurs after the above treatment, aeration of the middle ear cleft until spontaneous resolution takes place is achieved by introducing a small polyethylene tube (grommet) through a hole in the tympanic membrane. The tube is usually left in place for about six months until Eustachian tube function returns to normal.

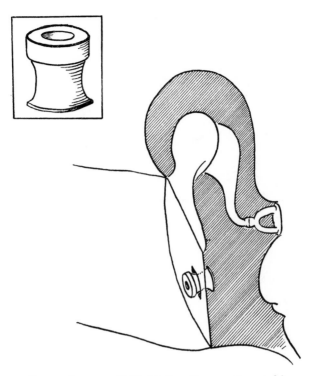

Fig. 11 Secretory Otitis Media. Grommet inserted in a
myringotomy incision. Inset—'Teflon' Grommet.

ACUTE OTITIS MEDIA

Acute otitis media is a common illness in infants and young school-
children, occurring more often during the winter season and especially
in children living in industrial areas.

Normal development of the middle ear and mastoid process

Acute otitis media usually occurs in a middle ear cleft which is normally pneumatised. The process of pneumatisation begins at birth.
Each time a child swallows the Eustachian tube opens and in this way
the air pressure on either side of the tympanic membrane is equalised.
As long as atmospheric pressure is maintained in the middle ear the air
cell system growing out from the mastoid antrum develops. This development continues until twelve years of age. The air cells are lined
with mucous membrane continuous with the rest of the middle ear
cleft. There is therefore a large air-containing space lined with mucous
membrane. In acute otitis media the lining of the whole space is
inflamed.

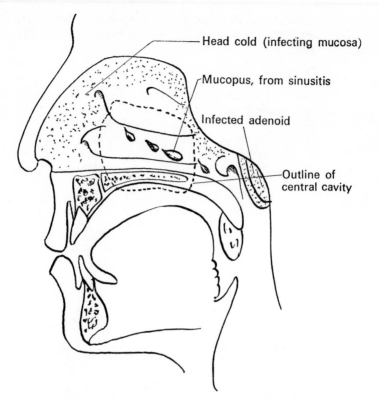

Head cold (infecting mucosa)

Mucopus, from sinusitis

Infected adenoid

Outline of
central cavity

Fig. 12 Acute otitis media. Sources of infection.

Sources of infection

Infection of the middle ear is usually secondary to disease of the nasopharynx. Firstly, the nasopharyngeal mucous membrane may become
infected during a cold and organisms are forced up the lumen of the
Eustachian tube by blowing the nose vigorously.

Secondly, an enlarged and infected pad of adenoid obstructs the
Eustachian opening so that the air in the middle ear is absorbed and
replaced by mucus. In turn, this becomes mucopus.

Thirdly, mucopus from the sinuses may flow into the post-nasal
space to infect the Eustachian tubes.

Route of infection

Organisms reach the middle ear from the nasopharynx and from the
external ear. They are usually streptococci, staphylococci or pneumococci.

Infection from the external ear follows water passing into the middle
ear through a perforation during swimming. The mucous membrane
becomes irritated and otitis media follows.

Generalised diseases such as measles or scarlet fever have been followed by severe otitis media, with destruction of the middle ear contents.

Pathology

The mucous membrane lining the Eustachian tube, middle ear and mastoid air cells becomes acutely inflamed. Mucopus collects in the middle ear and air cells. The tension in the middle ear increases, the tympanic membrane becomes inflamed, bulges and ruptures at its centre because of ischaemic necrosis. Mucopus is then discharged into the external ear. The drum heals and the Eustachian tube opens again.

The infection usually resolves with effective treatment and the middle ear returns to its normal appearance and function. Sometimes, however, the infection continues and complications follow.

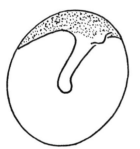

Redness of pars flaccida

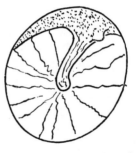

Increased vascularity of whole drum membrane

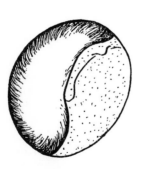

Bulging drum, with generalised suffusion

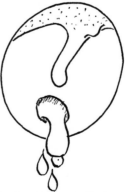

Perforation and discharge

Fig. 13 Stages in acute suppurative otitis media.

Clinical features

The symptoms are earache, discharge, deafness, malaise and fever.

Severe earache causes the child to awaken from sleep and scream with agony. A young baby may bang its head against the side of the cot or pull its ear.

General illness is common with a pyrexia of 101° F (38° C), vomiting, diarrhoea and sometimes a fit.

Discharge of mucopus from the ear brings instant relief from the earache. It may be the first symptom of ear disease. The mother finds a yellow stain on the child's pillow and looks at her child's ears.

Examination of the ear-drum shows signs of progressive inflammation in the middle ear. The margin of the tympanic membrane and the handle of the malleus are red. The whole tympanic membrane rapidly becomes very inflamed with loss of normal outlines; it bulges and ruptures with discharge of mucopus into the external canal. The discharge may pulsate and reflect light intermittently—the 'Lighthouse Sign' (Fig 13).

The mastoid process should be examined for tenderness or oedema. Efficient treatment during the early stages of acute otitis media prevents the disease from progressing. The perforation heals, regains its normal appearance and hearing is restored.

Investigations

Bacteriological examination of a swab of pus is helpful. The organisms and their sensitivity to antibiotic is shown, but the otitis media will be much improved by the time the report arrives.

Acute haemorrhagic otitis media progresses very rapidly. Vesicles arise in the outer layers of the drum. They may contain serum or blood. The patient suffers severe earache, followed by a blood-stained discharge.

Treatment

The child should be put to bed and encouraged to drink plenty of liquids. His earache must be relieved by Aspirin or Paracetamol. Antibiotics are given as soon as the clinical diagnosis has been made. Oral Penicillin 125 mg for 7 days will cure most patients with acute otitis media. Treatment must be continued until the tympanic membrane looks normal and hearing has been restored to normal.

Special measures

(i) *Aural toilet*

Careful removal of pus from the canal, followed by an antiseptic dressing helps to overcome the infection. It should be repeated daily until the ear has ceased to discharge.

(ii) *Myringotomy* (incision of drum)

Myringotomy is needed when there is a persistent collection of mucus or mucopus in the middle ear. These may cause continued deafness or a rapid recurrence of the otitis media. Both are relieved after the fluid has been removed from the middle ear.

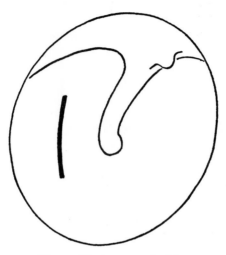

Fig. 14 Myringotomy incision.

Complications

1 Failure to resolve.
2 Rapid recurrence after earache has subsided.
3 Deafness, which may be temporary or permanent.
4 Spread of infection to the adjacent structures causing:

Acute mastoiditis
Facial nerve paralysis
Intra-cranial complications
Lateral sinus thrombosis

1. Failure to resolve

The antibiotic may have been taken for less than ten days, so that bacteria remain in the middle ear. The organisms may be resistant to Penicillin and the patient then requires a broad spectrum antibiotic.

2. Rapid recurrence

Rapid recurrence after complete resolution is probably due to infected adenoid or sinusitis reinfecting the middle ear through the Eustachian tube.

Adenoidectomy and antrum wash-outs treat two of the commonest causes of recurrent otitis media, but unfortunately a child living in bad social conditions may suffer further otitis media after the operation because of his unhygienic living conditions.

3. Deafness

(a) *Temporary deafness* due to mucus retained in the middle ear is relieved by aspiration through a myringotomy incision.

(b) *Permanent deafness* may follow repeated attacks of otitis media or a very severe infection because of damage to the ossicular chain or adhesions between the ossicles. The child then needs to use a hearing aid.

4. Spread of infection to adjacent structures
Acute mastoiditis

Acute mastoiditis is unusual since antibiotics have been used to treat otitis media. It still occurs in young babies who present with a tender swelling over the mastoid process. An older child is sent to hospital as an emergency, having suffered from acute otitis media for a week to ten days and no effective treatment has been given. The child is ill and has a mucopurulent discharge from the ear. There is a tender swelling over the mastoid process and the overlying skin is inflamed. A cortical mastoid operation is needed. The mastoid process is opened and the suppurating air cells are drained by removing their bony walls.

Facial nerve paralysis

Facial nerve paralysis is uncommon during acute otitis media. The facial nerve is usually protected by a bony wall during its passage through the middle ear but it may be exposed, due to absence of the wall in 10% of ears, and acute otitis media may then be followed by a facial nerve paralysis. The paralysis recovers completely as the otitis media resolves.

Intra-cranial complications and lateral sinus thrombosis

Labyrinthitis, brain abscess and lateral sinus thrombosis may follow acute mastoiditis. They will be discussed in Chapter Five.

Chapter Five
Chronic diseases of the middle ear cleft

Chronic suppurative otitis media causes a middle ear to discharge for many years. The two varieties of this disease are simple and serious chronic otitis media.

SIMPLE CHRONIC OTITIS MEDIA

Pathology
Recurrent otitis media destroys the pars tensa and the ossicles, the extent of destruction depending on the severity and frequency of the ear infections. The long process of the incus suffers earliest due to its poor blood supply. These patients never develop serious complications.

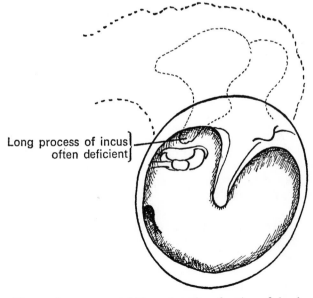

Long process of incus often deficient

Fig. 15 Large, central, kidney-shaped perforation of simple chronic otitis media.

Clinical picture

The patient complains of increasing deafness, recurrent discharge and occasionally earache. Pain is rare, but may follow water getting into the middle ear.

A large perforation of the pars tensa is present, exposing the promontory and the oval and round windows. Occasionally it is possible to see the opening of the Eustachian tube. The handle of the malleus often remains and the perforation is then kidney-shaped. The ear discharges mucopus during re-infections of the middle ear, but is dry in between. In this type of chronic otitis media the perforation is always in the centre of the tympanic membrane.

The upper respiratory tract must be examined to exclude infection in the nose or sinuses.

Audiogram shows a conductive deafness varying in severity (See p. 153).
X-ray of the mastoids may show a sclerotic mastoid or a reduction in the number of cells.

Treatment

Prophylactic. The ear should be protected with a clean piece of cotton wool covered with Vaseline while bathing; recently Silicone ear drops have been found to be very useful.

Treatment of a discharging ear requires aural toilet, carefully carried out and repeated daily until the discharge has ceased. A dressing soaked in antiseptic is laid in the ear after it has been cleaned.

Closure of the perforation is desirable:

1 To allow the patient to swim.
2 To help the patient to join one of the armed services.
3 To improve a slight degree of deafness due to a central perforation. When the deafness is more severe and the incus has been destroyed, a tympanoplasty operation will be required. Here the surgeon reconstructs the ossicular chain, as well as the tympanic membrane.

The surgeon must ensure that the ear has been dry for at least three months and there is no infection in the nose or sinuses before undertaking a plastic operation to close the perforation.

Residual deafness may make the patient ask for a hearing aid, especially when both ears are involved.

SERIOUS CHRONIC SUPPURATIVE OTITIS MEDIA

Pathology

This type of disease occurs in a middle ear cleft which has failed to become pneumatised in early childhood. It is believed that the Eustachian tube fails to open properly, so that the air pressure is not equalised on either side of the drum. Because the middle ear air pressure is lower than the pressure in the external canal, the pars flaccida, being the weakest part of the tympanic membrane, is pushed into the attic, forming a pouch. Epithelium is shed from the superficial layer of the membrane, forming concentric rings which accumulate within the pouch. This mass of epithelial cells, known as a cholesteatoma, enlarges and by pressure perforates the outer attic wall to discharge foul pus. Secondary infection by bacteria from the external auditory canal

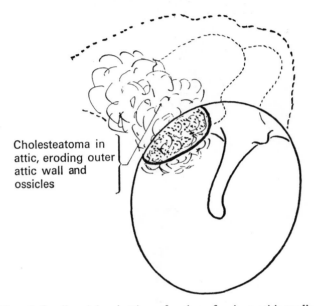

Cholesteatoma in attic, eroding outer attic wall and ossicles

Fig. 16 Small peripheral attic perforation of serious otitis media.

causes a persistent discharge and expansion of the cholesteatoma. As it continues to enlarge, the middle ear is invaded, causing destruction of the ossicular chain, the roof of the middle ear may be eroded and an intra-cranial complication result, or spread medially may involve the labyrinth and facial nerve.

Sometimes bacteria entering the middle ear through an attic perforation start an insidious chronic inflammation involving the bony margin of the tympanic ring or one of the ossicles, so that granulation tissue starts to grow.

Prolonged infection causes the granulation to grow and an aural polyp is formed.

To summarise, in this type of disease there is a perforation of the pars flaccida, associated with a cholesteatoma in the attic portion of the middle ear and a non-pneumatised mastoid process. Complications occur in this disease because of infection caused by erosion of surrounding vital structures by expansion of the cholesteatoma.

Clinical picture

The patient suffers from recurrent discharge and deafness. As the disease progresses, earache and vertigo may occur, presaging a serious complication. The ear is full of a foul discharge, which must be removed before the drum can be examined.

A perforation is seen in the pars flaccida or the margin of the posterosuperior quadrant of the tympanic membrane. The perforation may be

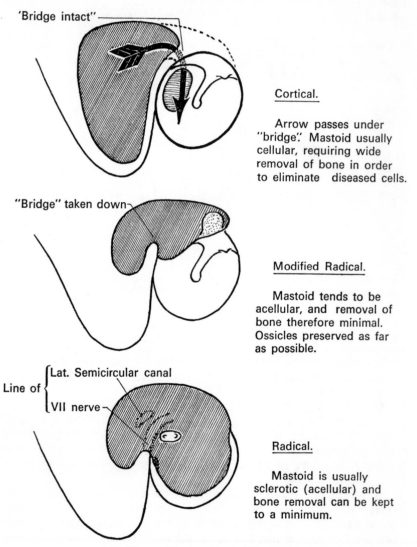

'Bridge intact'

Cortical.

Arrow passes under "bridge". Mastoid usually cellular, requiring wide removal of bone in order to eliminate diseased cells.

"Bridge" taken down

Modified Radical.

Mastoid tends to be acellular, and removal of bone therefore minimal. Ossicles preserved as far as possible.

Line of { Lat. Semicircular canal
VII nerve

Radical.

Mastoid is usually sclerotic (acellular) and bone removal can be kept to a minimum.

Fig. 17 Types of mastoid operation.

seen to be discharging white scales, or an aural polyp may be seen as a red pedunculated swelling attached to the bony margin. The polyp often bleeds when touched and pressure on it may be transmitted to an exposed labyrinth, causing the patient to become giddy.

Investigations
Audiogram shows a conductive deafness of varying severity.
X-ray of the mastoids. The mastoid is sclerotic, i.e. contains no air cells, and there may be a cavity in the bone due to erosion by cholesteatoma.

Treatment
The otologist tries to give the patient a safe ear which is dry and to preserve as much hearing as possible.

1 *Examination of the ear with a microscope* under general anaesthetic allows cholesteatoma to be removed from the canal. The patient then attends for daily aural toilet and his progress is supervised at weekly intervals. A further examination is needed if the discharge continues.

2 A mastoid operation is advised when this has failed, i.e. when the ear fails to remain dry. The principle of this operation is to remove the cholesteatoma and to make the mastoid antrum, the attic, middle ear and external auditory meatus into one cavity allowing easy access for toilet and removal of any persistent cholesteatoma. A radical mastoid operation is necessary when the ear is very deaf. The malleus and incus having been destroyed by chronic infection, it is best to remove the remnants.

A modified radical mastoid operation may suffice if the hearing is good, the disease limited to the attic region and the ossicles are intact.

The disease in the mastoid process is removed, followed by removal of the outer attic wall to enter the attic and middle ear. In a radical mastoid the remains of the drum and all the contents of the middle ear are removed except the stapes.

In a modified radical mastoidectomy the middle ear contents are left.

After a mastoid operation the patient is left with a cavity instead of an external canal and middle ear. He must attend an otological clinic at weekly intervals until the cavity has healed and later, every six months for removal of wax. Failure to do this allows the cavity to become filled with wax, causing labyrinthine irritation.

Recent advances in treating chronic suppurative otitis media
Otologists have tried to remove disease completely from the mastoid and middle ear whilst preserving the posterior bony canal wall. The

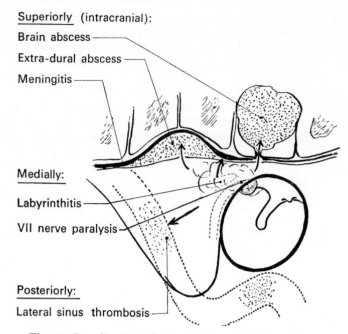

Superiorly (intracranial):
Brain abscess
Extra-dural abscess
Meningitis

Medially:
Labyrinthitis
VII nerve paralysis

Posteriorly:
Lateral sinus thrombosis

Fig. 18 Complications of serious otitis media, according to
direction of spread.

operation is known as the combined approach mastoid. The mastoid and attic explored and middle ear entered across the front of the facial nerve from behind. Access is restricted, disease may surround the ossicles and infiltrate the bone making complete removal difficult. The continuity of the ossicular chain is restored using an incus or cartilage homograft and the perforation of the drum closed with a graft of temporalis fascia.

The operation may take 4–5 hours to complete but residual cholesteatoma may grow to cause recurrence of the discharge. Most olologists have therefore abandoned it.

Complications of chronic serious suppurative otitis media

Intra-cranial complications are usually the result of direct spread of infection from the ear to the middle or posterior cranial fossae. Infection may enter through the labyrinth or by thrombosis of the veins between the middle ear and the meninges. The common intra-cranial complications are extra-dural abscess, meningitis and brain abscess.

Extra-dural abscess is a collection of pus between the tegmen and the dura. It may be so large that the dura is displaced, but remains intact.

The patient has had a discharging ear for many years but has not asked for advice. It becomes very painful and he may suffer severe headaches. The ear shows signs of serious chronic suppurative otitis media and there may be a tender swelling over the temporal region. Immediate admission to hospital is necessary and a course of Penicillin 500 000 units six-hourly by intramuscular injection started. A mastoid operation is performed as soon as possible, the abscess is drained and a radical mastoid operation completed.

Meningitis is a diffuse infection of the sub-arachnoid space. The patient suddenly becomes very ill with severe headache, vomiting and pyrexia. He is very restless at the onset, but soon loses consciousness and cannot be roused. The classical physical signs of meningitis soon appear: increasing stiffness of the neck, photophobia, a positive Kernig's sign and brisk reflex responses.

The diagnosis is confirmed by lumbar puncture. The cerebro-spinal fluid looks turbid and its pressure is increased. The protein concentration is raised, but the glucose and chloride are reduced. The cell count is increased to 100–10 000 polymorphs per cm^3 and organisms may be found in the stained film.

It is vital to start treatment immediately. Massive doses of soluble Penicillin are given by intramuscular injection, 1 million units every two hours. Penicillin is injected into the spinal theca, 10 000 units daily. Sulphadiazine G2 every four hours is needed to overcome the massive infection. Intramuscular Penicillin and Sulphadiazine should be continued for two weeks, but intrathecal Penicillin discontinued after three days. Intravenous fluids are also required. A radical mastoid operation is performed when the meningitis has settled down.

Brain abscess. This usually involves the temporal lobe and rarely the cerebellum. The patient develops severe headache, vomiting and drowsiness. There may be no abnormal signs in the central nervous system in the early stages. A right-handed person with an abscess in his left temporal lobe may have difficulty in naming familiar objects (nominal aphasia). Later, signs of pyramidal tract involvement are found.

The patient must be referred to a neuro-surgeon for aspiration of the abscess through a burr hole in the skull. A radical mastoid operation is performed when the abscess has settled down.

Labyrinthitis is the commonest complication of serious chronic suppurative otitis media. The labyrinth is infected through a fistula in the lateral semicircular canal or through the oval window by erosion of a cholesteatoma. The infection passes into the membranous labyrinth with destruction of the cells in the cochlear and vestibular organs.

The patient suffers from severe vertigo and vomiting. These are increased by movement of his head. He is pyrexial and generally unwell. His eyes show fine horizontal nystagmus and the vertigo may be increased by pressing on the diseased ear (fistula sign).

Immediate admission to hospital is necessary. A course of Penicillin by injection is begun (500 000 units every six hours) and Avomine by mouth 25 mg twice a day. A radical mastoid operation is performed next day to remove the cholesteatoma.

Facial nerve paralysis results from invasion of the nerve by cholesteatoma in the middle ear or mastoid process. A lower motor neurone paralysis develops which may become complete if neglected.

An immediate radical mastoid operation is necessary. The facial nerve is often surrounded by cholesteatoma, or acutely inflamed due to absence of its bony covering. Great care must be taken during the mastoid operation to avoid further damage to the nerve.

Lateral sinus thrombosis follows an abscess around the lateral sinus. The wall becomes infected with granulations on its surface and clot inside the lumen. Emboli may break off and pass into the bloodstream after the clot has become infected.

It is usually diagnosed during a mastoid operation for an acute flare-up of a chronic otitis media. Occasionally such a patient presents with swelling over the occiput. Pyaemic abscesses in the lung are rare nowadays.

The patient requires a radical mastoid operation.

Chapter Six
Deafness in adults

Deafness in both ears of an adult is a serious disability affecting the patient and his friends, but deafness involving one ear is not a serious disability provided the patient learns to use his good ear.

PHYSIOLOGY OF HEARING
Sound waves are collected by the auricle and pass along the canal to the tympanic membrane. The pars tensa vibrates in response to sound waves which are then conducted through the malleus and incus to the stapes. The stapes footplate articulates with the oval window and beneath it lies the utricle and saccule surrounded by perilymph. Movement of the stapes footplate causes sound waves to be conducted through the oval window to move the endolymph. This movement stimulates the delicate hair cells of the cochlea and from these cells impulses pass along the fibres of the auditory nerve to reach the auditory cortex in the superior temporal gyrus on both sides of the brain. Each hair cell is thought to respond to a specific frequency of sound.

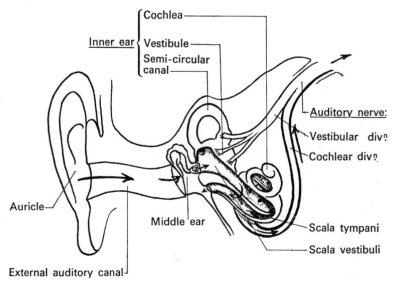

Fig. 19 Conduction of sound through the ear.

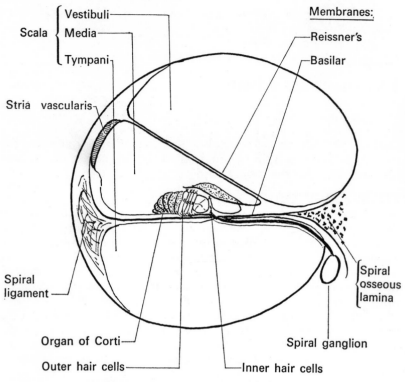

Fig. 20 Cross section through cochlea.

The ratio of effective surface area of the pars tensa to the stapes footplate is 14:1. The mechanical advantage gained from the leverage of the long handle of malleus acting through the incus onto the tiny stapes is 1·3 to 1 so that the sound-pressure transformation gain across the middle ear is 18·3 to 1. Therefore, destruction of the drum or part of the ossicular chain causes deafness by removing the mechanism of sound pressure transformation.

The cause of deafness may lie in the external, middle or inner ear.

CONDUCTIVE DEAFNESS

Conductive deafness is due to interference with the conduction of sound from the auricle to the oval window. For an audiogram of conductive deafness see p. 153.

Causes of conductive deafness in the external ear

  1 Wax.

  2 Chronic external otitis causing the canal to be filled with pus and debris. Sometimes the skin lining the canal becomes very swollen and conductive deafness results.

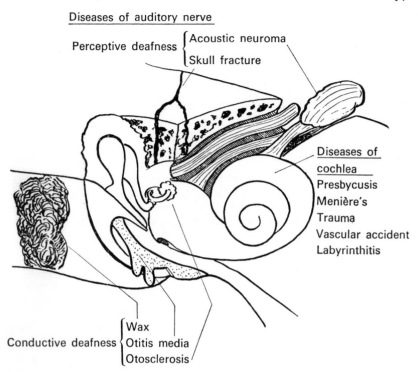

Diseases of auditory nerve

Perceptive deafness { Acoustic neuroma / Skull fracture

Diseases of cochlea
Presbycusis
Menière's
Trauma
Vascular accident
Labyrinthitis

Conductive deafness { Wax / Otitis media / Otosclerosis

Fig. 21 Common causes of deafness.

Causes of conductive deafness in the middle ear

Infections

  (a) Acute suppurative otitis media.

  (b) Acute secretory otitis media may follow a cold, acute sinusitis, chronic sinusitis or may occur in a patient with a carcinoma of his post-nasal space. The Eustachian orifice is oedematous, the tube becomes blocked, air is absorbed from the middle ear and fluid effuses into it from the mucosa.

    In these patients bubbles of fluid may be seen behind the tympanic membrane. A fluid level which alters with the position of the head, a slate-blue discoloration or a yellow discoloration resembling drops of oil on the surface of the tympanic membrane may also be seen.

  (c) Chronic suppurative otitis media either of the simple or serious type destroys part of the sound-conducting mechanism and so causes deafness.

Otosclerosis is a disease of the bony labyrinth. The normal Haversian bone is replaced by vascular bone laid down irregularly and which becomes sclerotic later. Involvement of the oval window by otosclerosis causes fixation of the stapes footplate thus preventing sound waves reaching the inner ear. The whole footplate is encroached on until it is a mass of sclerotic bone.

Several members of a family may be affected by this disease. Females suffer more often than males and successive pregnancies cause the disease to progress. The tympanic membranes are normal despite the patient being severely deaf, and an audiogram shows a severe conductive deafness.

Trauma to the middle ear may follow syringing of hard wax, a head injury or an unskilled attempt to remove a foreign body from the ear. The tympanic membrane may be perforated and the incus dislocated from its articulation with the head of the stapes. Thus the continuity of the ossicular chain is interrupted and deafness results. Less severe injuries cause bleeding into the middle ear space; the deafness is temporary and improves after the blood has been absorbed.

TREATMENT OF CONDUCTIVE DEAFNESS

Wax is removed by syringing after it has been softened.

Acute suppurative otitis media and *acute secretory otitis media* have been dealt with in Chapter Six.

Otosclerosis. The deafness may be relieved by the patient wearing a hearing aid or undergoing a stapedectomy operation. The decision rests entirely with the patient who should never be persuaded to undergo an operation, because otosclerosis is not a fatal disease. A hearing aid may irritate the skin and start an external otitis. It will amplify all sounds so that background noises are heard and can be very annoying.

A stapedectomy is always performed on the worst ear. If successful the operation restores hearing immediately. Vertigo may be troublesome immediately after operation, but improves with Avomine.

Chronic suppurative otitis media involving both ears causes a serious degree of conductive deafness. Operations to remove the offending disease have been outlined in a previous chapter. It may be possible to reconstruct the ossicular chain using a homograft to replace the incus and to reconstruct the tympanic membrane with a graft of temporalis fascia. Many patients continue to be deaf despite the operation to reconstruct the middle ear, so that a hearing aid is required.

SENSORY-NEURAL DEAFNESS

Sensory-neural deafness is the result of disease of the cochlea or of the auditory nerve or brain. For an audiogram of sensory-neural deafness see p. 153.

A patient suffering from sensory-neural deafness in both ears complains that he is unable to understand what people are saying. He can hear a noise but all the words are 'jumbled up', causing him to be very confused. An invitation to a social gathering is very embarrassing because he cannot understand what is being said, but talking to another person alone in a quiet room is possible. Shouting increases his confusion and he prefers people to speak slowly and distinctly. The common diseases affecting the cochlea are:

Degenerative. *Presbycusis* or deafness in old age is due to degeneration of the sensitive hair cells. It is the commonest cause of perceptive deafness.

Menière's disease. The endolymphatic canal becomes distended with fluid, causing destruction of the hair cells. The reason for this disease is still unknown; it may cause bilateral perceptive deafness.

Trauma. Exposure to high-pitched loud noises for a prolonged period destroys the cochlear hair cells. Boiler-makers, artillerymen firing heavy guns and 'Pop group' artists are especially prone to such an injury. Direct injury to the inner ear by fracture of base of skull involving the petrous temporal bone also destroys the inner ear.

Vascular accidents. Many patients suddenly develop a complete perceptive deafness for no apparent reason. It usually involves one ear and is thought to be due to obstruction of the blood supply to the inner ear.

Infective causes. Infection of the inner ear from cholesteatoma causes a suppurative labyrinthitis with total destruction of the inner ear. Mumps virus also has the same effect.

Sensory-neural deafness due to disease of the auditory nerve is usually unilateral. It may be due to injury or to a tumour causing pressure on the auditory nerve. The otologist has to decide whether a patient with unilateral sensory-neural deafness is suffering from disease of the cochlea or of the auditory nerve. A special audiogram (Loudness Balance, Bekesy, etc.) helps in the differential diagnosis.

TREATMENT OF SENSORY-NEURAL DEAFNESS

1 *Prophylactic.* People working near loud noises should protect their ears by wearing ear defenders. Large industrial firms should supply them to their employees and they should also measure the noise level at the site of work and when excessive, apply damping devices to the offending machines.

2 *Treatment of the deaf patient.* Once a patient has developed a total sensory-neural deafness it is impossible to restore his hearing. If the deafness is not profound, the patient will derive some benefit from a hearing aid. However, the principal problem in a patient with this type of deafness is often loss of discrimination; a hearing aid merely amplifies sound, including background noises, so that loss of discrimination is not helped —indeed, a hearing aid may even make matters worse.

Chapter Seven
Vertigo

DEFINITION
Vertigo is a sensation of abnormal movement of the surroundings in relation to the patient or of the patient in relation to his surroundings; suddenly everything spins round or moves up and down in front of him. This is often followed by vomiting, sweating and collapse, but never loss of consciousness. Other symptoms of ear disease are often present.

CAUSES
The following ear disorders may cause vertigo:

Menière's disease
Injury to the ear
Positional vertigo
Labyrinthitis—epidemic or secondary to chronic otitis media

Vertigo may also be caused by disease of the acoustic nerve, cerebellum, and the cardio-vascular system.

Menière's disease
The aetiology of this disease is unknown. Excessive fluid and salt intake, overwork and emotional upsets are possible causes.

The membranous labyrinth is dilated, with destruction of the sensory cells in the ampullae and cochlea. The disease usually involves one ear, but the opposite side may be affected later.

The patient is usually middle aged and suffers a sudden onset of severe *vertigo*, accompanied by nausea and *vomiting*. The attack lasts several hours, but he has to stay in bed for two or three days. Return to work is delayed because the patient is unsteady while walking and lacks self-confidence. The vertigo can recur after a complete remission which may be several months or only a few days. The patient becomes deaf during an attack, but his hearing recovers in the remission; he also complains of *tinnitus* in the affected ear, often worse before or during an attack. Unfortunately, many patients become progressively deaf as the disease progresses.

Trauma
A head injury is often followed by troublesome vertigo. A labyrinth

may be destroyed by a fracture of the base of skull, but in less severe injuries is disorganised temporarily.

A patient may be giddy soon after a mastoid or a stapedectomy operation during which the stapes footplate is disturbed, causing irritation of the inner ear. The vertigo usually lasts a short time only.

A mastoid cavity should be inspected regularly. Failure to do this allows the cavity to become filled with wax and so irritate the labyrinth.

Labyrinthitis

Viral labyrinthitis often occurs as an epidemic. The patient becomes ill with vertigo and vomiting. There are no other symptoms of ear disease. It is a short illness which keeps the patient in bed for about ten days. Recovery is rapid and there are no after-effects.

Mumps also causes labyrinthitis, but the patient may be left with residual nerve deafness.

Suppurative labyrinthitis is a complication of attic cholesteatoma after it has invaded the inner ear. The membranous labyrinth is destroyed and the ear made totally deaf. Meningitis follows occasionally.

The patient has suffered from a discharging ear for many years. He has not asked for help from an otologist because the ear has not been painful. Suddenly, he becomes very ill with severe vertigo, vomiting and headache.

The ear shows signs of serious chronic suppurative otitis media, and the eyes show horizontal nystagmus.

The patient must be admitted to hospital immediately. Penicillin 250 000 units six-hourly is given by intramuscular injections and Avomine 25 mg six-hourly, given by mouth. He will need to undergo a radical mastoid operation urgently to remove the cholesteatoma.

Positional vertigo

The patient complains of attacks of vertigo lasting a few *seconds*, brought on by moving the head or bending down. The patient does not suffer from earache, discharge or deafness.

Examination of the upper respiratory tract shows normal findings. The audiogram and caloric test are normal, but a sudden sharp movement of the head backwards may bring on vertigo and nystagmus.

The cause of positional vertigo is unknown. It has been suggested that it is due to a disorder of the utricle, others have blamed osteoarthritis of the cervical spine.

Most patients improve spontaneously after two or three months. When the patient is suffering from severe arthritis in the neck a cervical collar will help considerably.

ACOUSTIC NEUROMA

Acoustic neuroma is a benign tumour growing from the sheath of the auditory nerve. It may arise close to the origin of the nerve at the pons, along the course of the nerve in the posterior cranial fossa or in the internal auditory canal. The tumour grows very slowly and involves the auditory nerve, the facial nerve and later the cerebello-pontine angle.

The patient suffers from a slowly progressive deafness in one ear. He also becomes unsteady on his feet, but *rarely* suffers from episodes of severe vertigo. In advanced cases he experiences symptoms of raised intracranial pressure, i.e. headache, vomiting.

Examination of the upper respiratory tract shows normal findings apart from perceptive deafness in one ear. There may be horizontal nystagmus, loss of corneal sensation or slight facial nerve paralysis. A lumbar puncture should be carried out as the concentration in protein is often raised considerably.

Treatment depends on the size and site of the tumour. A large tumour growing in the cerebello-pontine angle requires removal by a neuro-surgeon. These operations have a high mortality rate. Complete removal of the tumour may be complicated by facial nerve paralysis. A small tumour growing in the canal can be removed by operating through the mastoid and entering the internal auditory canal by removing the semicircular canals.

INVESTIGATIONS

History

A description of an attack will help to confirm that the patient is suffering from vertigo.

Routine questions used on patients with ear disease should be asked, i.e. deafness, earache, discharge and tinnitus.

Details of fluid and salt intake, smoking habits, hours spent at work, head injuries and emotional upsets are useful in assessing contributory factors.

Examination

1 *General examination* of the upper respiratory tract, bearing in mind the possibility of attic cholesteatoma.

2 *Special examination of ears and labyrinth* when there is no evidence of chronic otitis media:

(i) Examination of the eyes for nystagmus.

(ii) An audiogram to assess hearing. Perceptive deafness is usual in patients with Menière's disease.

(iii) X-ray each mastoid to demonstrate the internal auditory meatus.

(iv) A caloric test of labyrinthine function. Cold water (20° C) is run into one ear. The underlying labyrinth is stimulated and the eyes react by showing horizontal jerking movements (nystagmus). The length of time the nystagmus lasts is measured. This is repeated on the opposite side—a normal response is for the nystagmus to last for two minutes. In Menière's disease there may be no response. Recently the duration of nystagmus has been recorded by electro-nystagmography. This gives an accurate record of the response.

(v) A neurologist's opinion to exclude disease of the central nervous system.

TREATMENT OF PATIENTS SUFFERING FROM VERTIGO DUE TO MENIÈRE'S DISEASE

During the acute phase the patient should be put to bed and given Avomine 25 mg six-hourly. When the vertigo and vomiting are severe, the patient's admission to hospital may be necessary. Promethazine (Phenergan) 25 mg and Chlorpromazine 1·25 mg by intramuscular injection, repeated every 6 hours for 24 hours, will control severe vertigo and vomiting.

During the quiescent phase the patient is advised to take these following precautions:

1 Reduce his fluid intake to three cups of liquid each day.
2 Stop taking salt with his food.
3 Stop smoking.
4 Stop over-working.

The majority of patients improve with these measures. There remains a small number of patients whose vertigo recurs and an operation is necessary on the ear responsible for the vertigo.

Where the patient has good hearing, an operation to relieve vertigo yet preserve hearing is advised.

1 *Myringotomy and insertion of grommet* into the ear with least hearing, will often give relief from recurrent vertigo. Eustachian obstruction is thought to be responsible for the pathology in the inner ear. The grommet acts as a secondary Eustachian tube allowing adequate aeration of the middle ear. It should be left in for a minimum of 3 months.

2 *Decompression of Saccus endolymphaticus* to reduce the pressure on the membranous labyrinth will relieve vertigo. The sac lies in contact with dura of the posterior fossa. It is approached through the mastoid but identification is difficult and the operation is not popular.

3 *Ultrasonic destruction* of the labyrinth leaving the cochlear intact has also been tried but has been abandoned by most otologists.

When one ear is severely deaf and is causing recurrent vertigo it should be destroyed by removing the membranous labyrinth. The patient is completely relieved of his vertigo by this operation and the loss of his residual hearing in the affected ear causes no distress.

Chapter Eight
Symptoms and signs of nasal disease

FUNCTION OF THE NOSE

The nose is an organ used to warm and moisten the air we breathe, as well as to smell and taste food which we prepare to eat. It adds resonance to the voice.

When the function of the nose is disturbed by disease the effects of the dysfunction may be local and general. It is therefore essential to examine the patient as a whole before proceeding to the inspection of the nasal cavities, sinuses and post-nasal space.

SYMPTOMS

Nasal obstruction

The commonest symptom of nasal disease is nasal obstruction—or inability to draw sufficient air through the nose to supply the oxygen requirements of the body. Since an inadequate supply of oxygen is incompatible with everday life the patient compensates by opening his mouth to a greater or lesser extent. The first objective evidence of nasal obstruction therefore is usually that the patient is breathing through the mouth. Mouth breathing may have been present for a short time or a long time. Short-term nasal obstruction in an adult will usually be associated only with a slight opening of the mouth and a 'nasal' voice.

Long-term nasal obstruction originating in early childhood will probably be associated with gross mouth breathing. The nose will be shorter in length relative to the size of the face than in a normal adult. The upper lip is short and the incisor teeth exposed to view. The palate is 'high arched' and narrow. This leads to overcrowding of teeth in the alveolar arch which are displaced and do not occlude properly with the lower jaw.

The anterior nares are small. The baby's instinct is to breathe through his nose. As his body enlarges an increasing muscular effort is required to draw sufficient air through the nasal cavities into the lungs. This requirement is PHYSIOLOGICAL and it leads to the proper development of the thoracic cage and the upper jaw. Due to this considerable effort

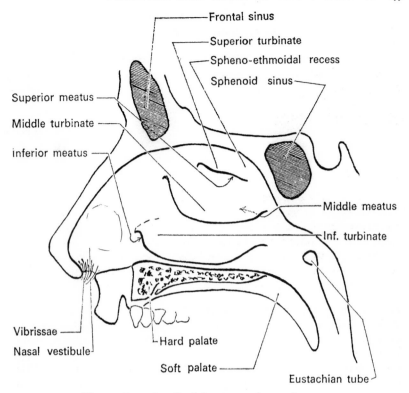

Fig. 22 Lateral wall of the nose and nasopharynx.

the nasal cavities enlarge as the body enlarges, the alveolar arches spread laterally and the teeth erupt in their proper site.

Mouth breathing on the other hand means that little or no muscular effort is required to breathe in adequate oxygen. As a result the nose falls into disuse. The nasal cavities fail to enlarge as the body enlarges. The alveolar arches do not expand and hence the teeth are crowded and irregular and the muscular development of the shoulder girdle is poor. Thus we see a round-shouldered, weedy, mouth-breathing individual, frequently with a stoop and generally poor skeletal development. This is known as the 'adenoidal facies'!

Nasal discharge

Discharge may be of mucus or mucopus, or blood. Following a fracture which involves the cribriform plate of the ethmoid there may also be a discharge of cerebrospinal fluid from the nose. In taking a history of nasal symptoms questions should be asked as to the manner of onset of the discharge, as to the side affected, whether it is getting better or worse, whether other symptoms, e.g. nasal obstruction or facial discomfort improves with the appearance of the discharge. If the discharge is of blood, enquiries relevant to the possible general causes of epistaxis (see Epistaxis, page 56) should be made. If the discharge is profuse and watery and associated with nasal irritation, then the enquiry should be directed towards the discovery of possible allergic factors.

Sneezing
Sneezing is a common symptom of nasal disease. Sneezing is a physiological mechanism whereby the nose can expel violently any foreign material which irritates the nasal mucous membrane. It is found in allergic rhinitis and when foreign bodies become lodged in the nasal cavities.

Loss of sense of smell
Every patient with some degree of generalised nasal congestion suffers from some diminution in the sense of smell. When the sense of smell is affected there will also be an effect upon the discrimination of flavour. It will be remembered that the tongue subserves the sensations only of sweet, sour and salt.

Headache and facial discomfort
This is not a very common symptom of nasal or sinus disease. It is, however, found in the acute infections which may complicate chronic sinusitis such as osteomyelitis, when it is accompanied by other signs of the disease. The classic sinus pain is worse in the morning. This is because the nasal mucous membrane is at its most congested in the morning due to the fact that the patient has been lying down for eight hours and the pull of gravity has been exerted equally over the whole body. Sinus pains tend to decrease as the day goes on.

EXAMINATION
Again before proceeding to the actual examination of the nasal cavities it is important to examine the external anatomy of the nose. Look for any irregularity in contour—a deviation of the tip to the right or the left. Any deformity of the nasal bones or any obvious swelling of either side. If the patient is elderly and there is a possibility of a malignant tumour having invaded the orbit a strabismus may be present and should be noted.

The anatomy of the nose is complicated and the student would be wise to revise it before examining the patient. The whole nasal cavity cannot be examined merely by the insertion of an appropriate nasal speculum into the nose and the shining of a light into the dark cavity beyond. Even after the nose has been sprayed with a vasoconstrictor solution (Adrenaline 1:1000) it may still not be possible to see beyond the middle meatus. Let us consider, therefore, the anatomy of what we are about to see.

The nasal vestibule is lined with skin in which are embedded hairs or vibrissae. Anteriorly or posteriorly, in the vestibule, fissures may appear in association with 'nose picking' and chronic infection. These fissures are extremely painful, particularly when the nares are dilated, and the examiner should, therefore, be extremely gentle in the use of a speculum. Beyond the vestibule the nasal cavity, lined with mucous membrane, widens out. To the lateral side we see the inferior turbinate shining and moist. Below it lies the inferior meatus, above it the middle meatus and above that, the middle turbinate. Medially lies the nasal septum. In the average nose this is all that can be seen. What then are we to look for? Three things are suggested:

1 Abnormality of the shape of the cavity.
2 Abnormality of the mucous membrane.
3 The presence of any abnormal structure or substance within, or within the wall of the cavity.

The nasal cavity may be narrowed either by twisting or 'deviation' of the nasal septum or by enlargement of a turbinate. In rare cases it may end as a blind pit. The septum may also be perforated low down anteriorly.

The mucous membrane may be of an abnormal colour or it may be producing abnormal secretions. Inflamed mucous membrane such as is seen in acute coryza or acute hay fever is fiercely congested and a deep red colour. Patients with a well-marked allergic rhinitis have a violet-coloured mucous membrane, and patients with a long-standing nasal allergy, the so-called chronic nasal oedema, have a very pale, swollen and wrinkled mucosa. Patients with emotional disturbances commonly have a cherry-coloured mucosa.

The mucus produced by the nose is generally adequate to keep the cavity moist but not excessively so. If mucus is over-produced and cannot be cleared, as may be seen in nasal allergy or in ciliary paralysis following one of the exanthemata such as measles, then mucus will tend to 'pool' on the floor of the nose. If, due to repeated infections, the number of mucous glands are reduced by fibrosis in the subepithelial tissues, then the passage of air tends to dry the mucus and it will then be found in small crusts lying on the mucous membrane.

There are two ways in which the nasal cavities may be inspected:

1 In infants and young children the nares tend to open forwards and all that is necessary is to tilt the tip of the nose up with the thumb and to direct a light into the nares. This has the added advantage that the nasal vestibule is not narrowed unnecessarily by the insertion of the blades of a speculum.
2 In older children and adults it is necessary to dilate the nares, which tend to open downwards, by the insertion of a two-bladed speculum of the Thudichum type.

There are many ways of holding the speculum. The student should adopt a method which gives him a good view and does not cause the patient discomfort.

Once the speculum is inserted the nasal cavity of one side is compared with the other side. Shape, size and type of mucous membrane are noted together with the presence or absence of foreign body, ulcer or tumour, polyp or discharge.

Having examined the anterior nasal cavities the surgeon always attempts to examine the post-nasal space. This is achieved by warming a small post-nasal mirror and passing it through the oropharynx and using it to reflect light from a head-mirror into the post-nasal space. The tongue is gently depressed with a Lacks tongue depresser. In this way the post-nasal space can be inspected piecemeal.

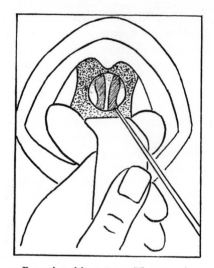

Fig. 23 Posterior rhinoscopy. The nasopharynx is examined a part at a time.

The post-nasal space is bounded anteriorly by the posterior choanae in which are seen the posterior ends of middle and inferior turbinates. In the midline lies the nasal septum. The most prominent feature on the lateral walls of the space are the Eustachian cushions, above which lie the fossae of Rosenmuller. The nasopharyngeal tonsil or adenoid hangs from the roof and posterior wall in children up to the age of twelve, and the floor is formed by the upper surface of the soft palate which is of course deficient posteriorly during quiet breathing.

The presence or absence of adenoids is noted. The nasal septum, the posterior end of which forms the medial boundary of each posterior choana, is found and followed upwards to the roof of the nose. Moving laterally across the roof the fossae of Rosenmuller are examined and then the Eustachian cushions. The presence or absence of polypi, ulcers or tumours and nasal discharge is recorded.

No clinical examination of the nose can be looked upon as complete until there has been some estimation of nasal function. An objective assessment of function is extremely difficult, but a rough estimate may be made by asking the patient to close his mouth and to breathe out through the nose. A shiny tongue depressor held beneath the nostrils will then show two areas of misting which can be compared for:

1 Size.

2 Speed of disappearance.

This is, of course, a measurement only of the expiratory tide and is of limited value.

It may also be necessary to assess the patient's subjective ability to detect certain smells. Generally speaking aromatic oils such as peppermint, eucalyptus or oil of wintergreen are used. Ammonia should not be used because it can cause reflex lacrimation by stimulation of the nasal rather than the olfactory mucous membrane.

INVESTIGATIONS

Frequently the surgeon is unable to make a diagnosis on the basis of a clinical examination alone. He may therefore call for radiographs of the paranasal sinuses. Two standard views are taken. For both views the tube is placed behind the patient. The antra are shown through the parietal bones in the occipito-mental (nose and chin) position. The ethmoids and frontals are demonstrated in the occipito-frontal (forehead and nose) view. Radiographs reveal the normal bony anatomy and may in addition show shadows within the cavities of the sinuses or nose. These shadows which are lighter than normal areas may only be interpreted in association with the history and clinical examination. In this way the presence of fluid or chronic inflammation may be established. Finally radiology may demonstrate osteoporosis in acute osteitis, osteosclerosis in chronic osteitis and erosion in malignant disease.

Chapter Nine
Injuries of the nose and deflected nasal septum

PATHOLOGY

The nose is one of the parts of the body which is frequently injured. The force causing the injury may be frontal or lateral, and the real importance of injuries occurring in this area is not so much in the resulting disfigurement as in the possibility of associated injuries to surrounding structures. Thus nasal disfigurement may be the most obvious abnormality, but a fracture of the middle third of the face may present a much more urgent problem. The clinical approach to the fractured nose becomes all-important.

The skin over the nasal bones is stretched tightly and there is very little subcutaneous tissue. Consequently it is likely that a blow on the nose will result in laceration of the skin and a compound fracture. Through the laceration infection may be introduced, and if there are any of the associated injuries mentioned above, the pathway for development of serious complications is there. It is therefore important that a routine is established for the management of this common injury. Frontal forces applied to the nasal bones cause them to splay laterally over the frontal processes of the maxillae. If these forces are sufficient, the nasal septum may be buckled and the cribriform plate of the ethmoid fractured. Through this fracture, C.S.F. may escape into the nasal cavity. Laterally directed blows tend to drive the nasal superstructure laterally across the face.

In addition to the fracture and possible laceration of the skin, there is usually rupture of a number of blood vessels, with which the nasal cavities are richly supplied. This leads to the rapid development of a haematoma, and there may be profuse bleeding from the nares (epistaxis). The volume of this bleeding may be such as to mask an underlying C.S.F. rhinorrhoea. The haematoma as it forms, increases the separation between the fragments of bone and if it is allowed to develop fully it will not be possible to stabilise the fragments in position after manipulation. This is important in deciding when to reduce the fracture.

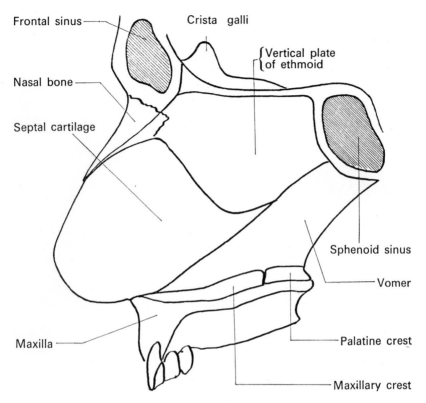

Fig. 24 Anatomy of nasal septum.

CLINICAL PICTURE

The patient with maxillo-facial injuries involving the nose usually reports to hospital with epistaxis and lacerations of the face and nose. He may also complain of a deformity of the nasal outline. He is unlikely to complain of anaesthesia of the cheek or teeth, although this symptom may indicate a more serious fracture of the maxilla with crushing of the infra-orbital nerve.

It may not be possible to get a clear view of what is going on in the nasal cavities because of profuse bleeding.

INVESTIGATION

If the patient is conscious at the time he is first seen, he should be asked whether he has at any time since the accident lost consciousness.

Before proceeding to examine the local condition a neurological assessment should be carried out. The function of each cranial nerve should be tested.

The external examination of the head should record:

(i) The nature and degree of deformity.

(ii) A careful description of the size and location of lacerations.

(iii) The presence or absence of suspected C.S.F. rhinorrhoea.

(iv) The presence or absence of anaesthesia over the face and teeth.

(v) Any abnormality of occlusion of the upper and lower jaws. In middle third fractures the upper teeth come to lie behind the lower.

(vi) The presence of trismus and/or blood in the external auditory meatus (associated with fractures of the glenoid fossa).

X-rays should be taken of the skull and nasal bones and the report placed in the case record.

TREATMENT

Detailed operative treatment is outside the scope of this book.

General treatment

In all but the most trivial fractures, the patient should be admitted to hospital and nursed in bed, sitting up. If the fracture is compound he should be given antibiotics and appropriate anti-tetanus prophylaxis. Any lacerations are sutured immediately. If there is malocclusion of teeth or anaesthesia of the teeth, the maxillo-facial surgeons must be consulted.

Local treatment

The fractured nasal bones should be reduced either before the haematoma has formed, i.e. within the first two hours after the injury, or after the haematoma has begun to absorb, i.e. after a week to ten days but not more. In all but the most trivial fractures the nose is placed in a plaster of Paris splint for ten days after reduction of the fracture. The patient should sleep in the splint for a further ten days.

DEVIATION OF THE NASAL SEPTUM

Aetiology

In almost everyone the two nasal cavities are of different size. In most cases this appears to be due to variation in the rate of growth of the two sides of the face. In many cases it appears that the narrowing is due to a deviation of the nasal septum causing a partial dysfunction of that side. The septum may be dislocated into one nasal cavity inferiorly as a result of a frontal blow on the nasal bones. In almost all children

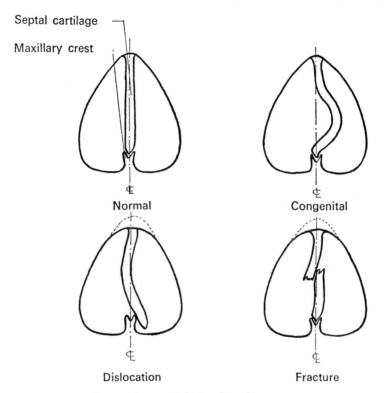

Fig. 25 Causes of deviated nasal septum.

with a cleft palate, there is a deviation of the nasal septum causing obstruction of one or other nares.

Pathology

Dislocations of the nasal septum may affect the anterior cartilaginous or the posterior bony parts of the septum. In anterior dislocations the whole vertical cartilaginous plate tends to be angled away from the sagittal plane and the nasal cavities may thus be obstructed. Posterior deviations usually take the form of bony spurs which protrude into the nasal cavity and may even press on the turbinates suspended from the lateral nasal wall. If the dislocations are gross, then the hollow created on one side of the septum may be filled by a compensatory hypertrophy of the middle or inferior turbinate on that side; if this does not take place, then the tide of air passing through that side of the nose will cause extreme drying of the mucus in the nose. This leads to atrophic changes in the ciliated epithelium of the mucous membrane.

Deviation of the septum may cause obstruction to the drainage of the paranasal sinuses. This may lead to important complications in the patient who develops an acute sinusitis or an acute exacerbation of a chronic sinusitis.

Clinical picture

The patient with a deviation of the nasal septum always complains of nasal obstruction. The difficulty experienced may be either on inspiration or expiration. Sometimes there is a complaint of headache or pain around the eye. The sense of smell is usually unimpaired.

Anterior dislocations of the septal cartilage are readily diagnosed by anterior rhinoscopy. The tip of the nose is gently raised by the examiner's thumb when the septum will be clearly seen projecting into the obstructed nostril.

Posterior deflections can often be seen only after the mucous membrane has been shrunken by the application of 1:1000 Adrenaline solution. The spurs can then be seen. The shrinking of the nasal mucous membrane is very important in the assessment of the patient with this condition. Resection of the septum will only benefit those patients whose noses are still obstructed after the mucosa has been shrunken.

After an anterior inspection of the nasal cavities, the post-nasal space should be examined in order to confirm that the posterior end of the septum lies in the midline, and that there is no evidence of choanal atresia.

Indications for operation

Deviations of the septum are extremely common, but very few of the patients with the condition need surgical treatment.

There are four main indications for surgery:

1 Total or subtotal obstruction of one nasal cavity by a bony or cartilaginous deflection.
2 Obstruction to the drainage of one of the paranasal sinuses.
3 As an operation of access to a bleeding point in cases of epistaxis.
4 As an operation of access to the patient's ethmoid or sphenoid sinuses.

Operative treatment

Two forms of operation are possible:

1 The cartilaginous and bony septum may be dissected away from the mucous membrane and then removed with punch forceps and mallet and gouge. This operation is called submucous resection of the septum.
2 The septum may be straightened by the division of its attachment to any laterally placed structure and the removal of any

redundant portion. This procedure is called septal repositioning. This is technically a more difficult procedure, but in selected cases it gives excellent results. It is the operation of choice for children because it does not interfere with the growth of the nose.

Chapter Ten
Epistaxis

DEFINITION
Epistaxis is a symptom or a sign. It seems that this should be said at the beginning of this chapter because all too often it is looked upon as a disease. Nose-bleeding is the result of some local or general disease in the body. While it is imperative to discover where the bleeding is coming from and to stop it, it is equally necessary to find and treat the cause. It has been said in the past that there are fifty-four separate causes for epistaxis. This may or may not be true but the mental effort required to learn the list of causes serves no useful purpose. What should be understood are the various mechanisms which may be at fault and which may result in nose-bleeding.

AETIOLOGY
Clearly the nose-bleeding is initiated by the rupture of a blood vessel in the nasal mucous membrane. The reason that the bleeding does not

	Local	General causes
Congenital	Telangiectasis	Haemophilia or other coagulation defect
Acquired Traumatic	Fractured nose Foreign body Nose-picking	Crush injury Fractured skull and/or Middle one-third of face
Inflammatory acute chronic	Acute rhinitis Sinusitis Chronic rhinitis, sinusitis Syphilis, tuberculosis Actinomycosis	Hay fever Exanthemata, glandular fever Pyaemia and septicaemia
Neoplastic	Benign haemangioma Carcinoma	Lymphosarcoma Leukaemias
Circulatory	Back pressure from enlarged adenoids	Hypertension
Blood dyscrasias		Purpuras Agranulocytosis

stop may lie in the bloodstream, the vessel wall or in the mucosa, lining the nose itself. There may be back pressure on the veins in the nasal mucosa. There may, for example, be some infection in the nasal cavity which irritates the mucosa. Although lists should be avoided where possible and be replaced by principles, some form of classification must be given.

This is NOT intended to be a comprehensive list of the causes of epistaxis but to serve to call to mind those investigations which may be required when once the epistaxis has been controlled.

CLINICAL PICTURE

Epistaxis is usually of sudden onset. The quantity lost may be small or large. The bleeding may come from one bleeding point or many, and may arise at the front, particularly Little's area, or at the back of the nose. The patient is always anxious if the bleeding has been sufficiently troublesome for him to have to summon a doctor. A great deal of blood may have been swallowed and the patient may vomit blood copiously. It is, therefore, necessary to have a routine for dealing with the situation. The first need is to stop the bleeding.

TREATMENT

The patient should be sat up on an examination couch and suitably draped in a protective mackintosh. A head-mirror or headlight and a good examination light are essential. It is also necessary to have a good nasal sucker. The nares are gently dilated with a nasal speculum and the clots sucked away. It may then be possible to see the actual bleeding point. That area from which bleeding commonly arises is on the nasal septum anteriorly just above the posterior end of the nasal vestibule. This is called 'Little's' area. If the bleeding is coming from Little's area a piece of cotton wool soaked in equal parts of Lignocaine 4% and adrenaline hydrochloride 1:1000 should be squeezed out and inserted into the nostril. The end of the nose should then be squeezed for a few minutes to bring pressure to the bleeding point. The wool can be removed after three or four minutes. This alone may be sufficient to control the bleeding, but it may recur once the vaso-constrictor effect has worn off. For this reason the bleeding point should be sealed by the application of a cautery. This can be either a chemical or an electric cautery. It may be necessary to deal with several bleeding points in this way.

However, not all epistaxis can be controlled in this way. In severe hypertension, in which the loss of blood may be a 'safety valve' mechanism it may be necessary to put pressure on the nasal mucosa. This can be done either by passing an inflatable bag into the nasal cavity and filling it with air or water or by the insertion of a nasal pack. Since most doctors may have to pack a nose at some point in their career the procedure will be described in detail.

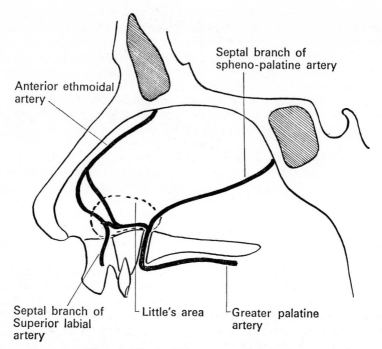

Anterior ethmoidal artery

Septal branch of spheno-palatine artery

Septal branch of Superior labial artery

Little's area

Greater palatine artery

Fig. 26 Blood supply of the nasal septum.

The average adult nasal cavity will hold about four feet (1·2 metres) of half-inch (13 mm) selvage gauze packing. For the purpose of packing an adult nose therefore, about eight feet (2·4 metres) of half-inch (13-mm) selvage gauze is required. If the pack is to remain *in situ* for any length of time it will act in the same way as any other foreign body and so either it should contain some anti-infective agent impregnated in the substance of the gauze or the packing must be covered by the exhibition of an appropriate antibiotic. What goes in has to come out, and unless the pack is suitably lubricated, removal may cause superficial damage to a debilitated mucosa and thus result in further bleeding. For this reason the ribbon gauze used should be impregnated either with Vaseline, in which case an antibiotic cover will be required, or with Bismuth Iodoform Paraffin Paste (B.I.P.P.).

The packing is introduced using Tilley's nasal dressing forceps. It is important that the pack is introduced in an orderly fashion so that the whole area of the nasal mucous membrane receives its pressure control. Figure 27 indicates how this should be done.

Both cut ends of the gauze should present at the anterior nares in order to prevent the loose ends from slipping into the nasopharynx where the irritation may cause retching leading to further bleeding. All four ends should be secured with a safety pin.

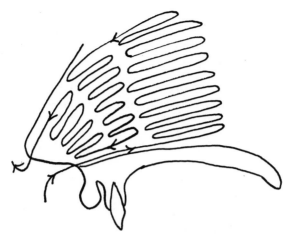

Fig. 27 Nasal packing in epistaxis.

The majority of cases of epistaxis can be controlled by these methods. If blood continues to flow down the nasopharynx it may be necessary to insert a post-nasal pack or even to tie off some part of the arterial supply, but such measures are outside the scope of this book as they are better carried out by those specially trained in the technique.

Once the bleeding has been brought under control it is important to assess the patient's general condition. Information is required about the following matters:

1 Is the patient shocked?
2 How much blood has been lost?

It may be difficult to provide an accurate answer to (2) until haemodilution has taken place. However, apart from a general clinical appraisal, half-hourly pulse counts and hourly blood pressures should be charted so that the response to treatment may be gauged. If the blood loss is thought to have been severe, blood samples should be taken for grouping and cross-matching and the laboratory alerted about the possible need for supplies.

The following investigations are required:

1 Full blood picture including haemoglobin, red and white cell counts and packed cell volume.
2 A nasal swab or post-nasal swab must be sent for culture.
3 Where there is no obvious general disease which could cause nose-bleeding, sinus X-rays should be ordered.

Second line of treatment
While the bleeding is being brought under control and the cause looked for, the patient should have complete *bed rest*. In order to

minimise any possible congestion of the mucous membrane which may occur from lying down he should be nursed *propped up* on a back-rest. Children are frequently in the prodromal stage of the exanthemata and are therefore best isolated.

When the nose is packed it has been taken out of service. The mouth will therefore be required to moisten and warm the air breathed in. This throws an extra burden on the mouth and it is particularly important to pay attention to oral hygiene. Mouthwashes and brushing of teeth should be carried out at frequent intervals during the day. Extra fluid must be provided (a) to replace that which has been lost, and (b) to lubricate the mouth. When the nose has been packed the patient will find it easier to take this fluid with a drinking straw. Whenever fluids are of particular importance to a patient the intake and output of fluid should be recorded on a chart so that a satisfactory fluid balance can be struck.

Drugs
Drugs may be needed for two purposes.

1 To allay the patient's anxiety and to make him more comfortable. In adults adequate doses of phenobarbitone are found to be the most useful. Morphia is contra-indicated because of the possibility of respiratory depression. In older children small doses of phenobarbitone are often helpful.

2 Drugs may be required to treat the cause or the effect of the epistaxis. Thus it may be necessary to prescribe antibiotics or agents to control the blood pressure or to deal with any abnormal blood condition.

If, after thorough investigation, no cause for the bleeding can be found, it should not be treated as an 'act of God' and the search abandoned. The patient should be referred to a physician for further investigation.

Chapter Eleven
The stuffy nose

DEFINITION
The title of this chapter is vague. The intention of the chapter is to throw light on that mysterious symptom 'catarrh' which sends so many patients to their doctor in despair.

Literally catarrh means 'that which falls from the nose' or nasal discharge. However, only rarely does the patient complaining of 'catarrh' mean that he is suffering from nasal or post-nasal discharge. The wise doctor runs the risk of being regarded as an ignoramus by his patient when he asks, 'What do you mean by catarrh?' The variety of answers obtained are surprising. In Lancashire, for example, one may be told 'Me nose is made up' by country people. Others mean nasal obstruction, nasal irritation, headache or sneezing. We have therefore to clarify what the patient means before we go any further with the matter.

As we get nearer to the twenty-first century, life becomes increasingly sophisticated. As the gateway through which air enters the body, the nose takes more than its share of the results of this sophistication. Thus, whereas in former times, smoke from the fire and pollen from grass, trees and flowers were almost the only problems with which the nose had to contend, nowadays each month adds to the chemical pollution of our environment. Huge power stations disseminate grit and sulphur dioxide over the land. Chemical products and fuel refineries discharge their waste into the atmosphere. As we go to work in the big cities we are engulfed in clouds of ill-controlled exhaust fumes from cars. Cosmetics are playing a more and more important part in our lives and all of these things can exert an irritant effect upon the nasal mucosa. These are the products of the twentieth century, but there have been three irritants for much longer than this which have caused chronic irritation of the lining of the nose in the past. These are DUST, ALCOHOL and TOBACCO. At this stage in our 'civilisation' as the tide of the former has swelled so the need for the latter appears to be on the increase. These effects are obvious and are well recognised. What is perhaps not so well understood is the effect of the internal environment upon the function of the nose. Only in the past twenty years have physicians realised that food allergies are not the only factor giving rise to nasal obstruction 'from within'. Certain drugs and hormone preparations are now well recognised as having nasal obstruction as a side effect and we are at last coming to realise that emotional and particularly sexual frustration may be associated with nasal obstruction every bit as disabling as perennial rhinitis.

HISTORY

Thus when a patient presents with 'catarrh' the doctor has to approach the problem in an orderly fashion. He has to answer the following questions.

1 Is there a local focus in the nose which is causing the symptom? This is what most patients believe.

2 Is the stuffiness due to some agent being inhaled?
  These may be—
  (i) Allergens—pollen, cosmetics, fungal spores, etc.
  (ii) Tobacco.
  (iii) Chemical fumes or suspensions.

3 Is the stuffiness due to an agent which has been swallowed?
  These may include—
  (i) Drugs—including alcohol.
  (ii) Food.

4 Is the stuffiness due to an inborn non-specific hypersensitivity? Chronic allergic rhinitis—vasomotor rhinitis.

5 Is the stuffiness due to emotional instability or sexual frustration?

In order to clarify the position an accurate history is essential. These questions should be put to the patient:

1 How long has the symptom been present?

2 Are one or both sides of the nose affected?

3 Is it getting better or worse?

4 Did the symptom begin with upper respiratory tract inflammation (a cold)?

5 Are there any of the following associated symptoms?
  (a) Headache.
  (b) Nasal discharge. If so, is it mucoid or mucopurulent, unilateral or bilateral?
  (c) Loss of sense of smell and taste.
  (d) Sneezing or irritation of the eyes and nose.

6 Does the symptom become worse at a particular time of the year or day?

7 Does the symptom become worse after taking particular food or drink?

8 Does the symptom become worse after contact with animals or birds?

9 Do the symptoms improve in another climate?

10 Is the occupation dirty?
11 How much is smoked?
12 How much alcohol is taken?

To obtain such a history takes time. However, it is time well spent, for it provides not only the answers to these all-important questions, it provides much interesting and valuable information about the patient and his habits from which it may be possible to form an opinion about the patient's emotional and domestic background. It is *most unlikely* that any patient would admit either to emotional instability or to sexual frustration. Such questions should not be put, therefore, until confidence in the doctor–patient relationship is firmly established.

EXAMINATION

The nose must now be examined and while this is going on the doctor is looking for some local structural or pathological defect which could produce the symptom. Such positive findings would include a local obstruction of the airway such as:

1 a foreign body
2 a deviation of the nasal septum or atresia
3 a purulent discharge
4 a nasal polypus
5 a neoplasm, either benign or malignant

The only one of the above conditions which does not *of necessity* require treatment is the deviation of the nasal septum. It may or may not be causing an obstruction. Unless it can be proved that it is, treatment should not be advised. All of the conditions require further investigation, which may include sinus X-rays, culture of a nasal swab, removal and histological examination.

If there is no obvious obstruction in the airway, then an assessment should be made as to whether the airway is narrowed by swelling of the mucous membrane. The following points are of value in the assessment of the condition of the mucous membrane:

1 The colour— (a) Red (seen in acute rhinitis and chronic rhinitis due to chemicals, alcohol, tobacco, drugs, etc.).
(b) Morello cherry-red (seen in emotional and sexual frustration).
(c) Violet (seen in vasomotor rhinitis and nasal allergy).
(d) Blue-grey (seen in long-standing nasal allergy).
2 What happens when the mucosa is shrunken down with a vaso-constrictor solution? Is there drainage of pus or an obvious bony irregularity of the septum?

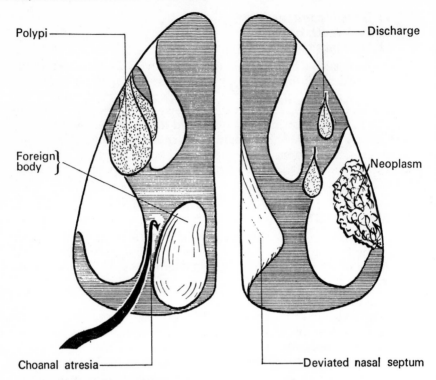

Polypi

Discharge

Foreign body

Neoplasm

Choanal atresia

Deviated nasal septum

Fig. 28 The stuffy nose. Local defects causing nasal obstruction.

INVESTIGATIONS
At this stage it is of value to have the following investigations carried out:

(i) X-rays of the sinuses.
(ii) Examination of the nasal mucus for eosinophils.

TREATMENT
If there is any doubt that the sinuses are radiologically clear, then the antrum should be washed out and any pus obtained sent for culture. If the wash-out is clear and the drainage good, then it seems probable that the patient is suffering from a chronic rhinitis of some form, the causes and treatment of which are shown in Figure 29.

Vasomotor rhinitis should be treated surgically when the symptoms are primarily obstructive and with anticholinergic drugs when the symptoms are of hyper secretion.

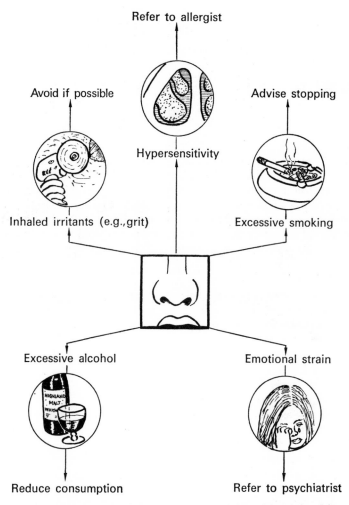

Fig. 29 Causes and treatment of chronic rhinitis without sinusitis.

Chapter Twelve
Nasal polypi

DEFINITION
Nasal polypi are areas of nasal mucous membrane distended with intercellular fluid and pulled down into the nasal cavity by gravity. This definition covers the large majority of polypi seen in practice. However, it is also important to bear in mind that areas of nasal mucous membrane may become distended by back pressure on the veins due to neoplasia in the nose and unilateral nasal polypi seen AT ANY AGE should be treated as potentially malignant until proved to be otherwise.

AETIOLOGY
Most nasal polyps appear to develop as a result of a hypersensitivity or atopic response in the nasal mucous membrane. Focal tissue damage in the mucosa leads to the overproduction of intercellular fluid and the tendency to polyp formation.

PATHOLOGY
The gross appearance of a benign nasal polyp resembles closely a skinned grape. It is normally attached to bone by a narrow pedicle from which it hangs down into the nasal cavity. On microscopic section no increase in the actual number of cells is seen but the cells are widely separated by intercellular fluid The covering mucous membrane is pseudostratified columnar epithelium. It may be possible to see many eosinophils in the substance of the polyp. Where the mass of the polyp causes obstruction to the drainage of a sinus there may be superadded infection. In rare cases infection may result in bacterial allergy and the polyp may form as a result of infection. They tend to recur.

SYMPTOMS AND SIGNS
Any mass hanging free within the cavity of the nose causes *nasal obstruction*. This is the prime symptom of nasal polyposis. The blockage may be so severe as to cause *loss of sense of smell*. Where the drainage of the sinuses is affected the patient may also complain of *headache* and *nasal discharge*. If the underlying cause is nasal allergy, then there may be complaints of nasal irritation and sneezing.

Benign nasal polypi resemble skinned grapes. They are usually bilateral and hang down from the region of the middle turbinate into

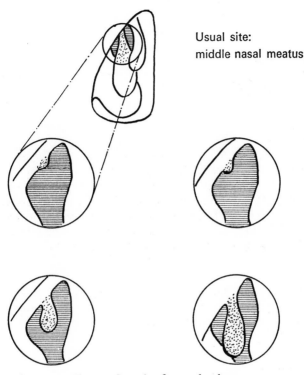

Usual site:
middle nasal meatus

Fig. 30 Genesis of a nasal polypus.

the lumen of the nose. When the drainage of the sinus has been prejudiced by the presence of the polyp the swelling may be bathed in pus. Innocent nasal polypi are not ulcerated, do not bleed and are not usually unilateral. They are not usually associated with gross enlargement or deformity of the external nose. If any of these signs are encountered the polyp should be regarded as potentially malignant and investigated as a matter of urgency.

INVESTIGATIONS

Since the polypi are causing nasal obstruction they will have to be removed. However, the obstruction may be not only to the airway but also to the paranasal sinuses. Infection may therefore be present in the sinuses. If the polypi are removed in the presence of unsuspected infection a secondary haemorrhage could occur. For this reason X-rays of the sinuses are taken and a nasal swab cultured before any surgery is undertaken. Once the polypi have been removed and sent for histological examination the patient should be referred to an allergist for investigation of the cause and for advice and treatment.

TREATMENT

Nasal polypi are removed under local or general anaesthesia by means of a nasal cutting snare. If the sinuses are infected drainage may be required and the procedure should be carried out under an antibiotic cover.

Antro-choanal polyp

This is a special type of nasal polyp which occurs more commonly in boys than girls and is seen in adolescents and young adults. It is associated with a congenital abnormality of the maxillary antrum in which the antrum develops from two buds rather than one. The polyp fills the cavity of the antrum and enlarges into the nasal cavity and ultimately comes to hang down into the post-nasal space. It is therefore 'dumb-bell shaped'. It is always unilateral. In the first instance it is customary to treat it by avulsion. However, it tends to recur and it must then be approached through the canine fossa and removed completely.

Chapter Thirteen
Acute sinusitis

DEFINITION
Acute sinusitis is an acute inflammation of the mucosa of any or all of the paranasal sinuses. The inflammation may be suppurative or non-suppurative.

AETIOLOGY
Acute sinusitis usually results from a secondary bacterial infection of an acute rhinitis. The lining of the nose and sinuses are in continuity and inflammation spreads easily from one area to another. The bacteria usually cultured from the pus include streptococci, pneumococci and staphylococci. However, acute sinusitis may also result from trauma, e.g. fractures of the maxillae and frontal bones, from foreign bodies in the nose and from dental sepsis. Attacks may also be provoked by diving into water 'feet first' without pinching the nose.

PATHOLOGY
The pathology of acute sinusitis is similar to the pathology of an acute inflammation of any epithelial surface, modified only by the local anatomy. In the case of the paranasal sinuses the disease is modified by the following factors:
  (i) The mucosa lines an air-containing cavity.
 (ii) The drainage ostium of the sinuses is small and tends to become sealed off with fibrin early in the inflammatory process.
(iii) The rich blood supply of the area and the proximity to the brain and meninges makes the development of intracranial complications a danger.

Sequence of events
The inflammatory reaction goes through all its characteristic phases. Dilatation of the capillaries, slowing of the bloodstream with pouring out of fibrin and exudate, and the migration of the leucocytes through the walls of the blood vessels to form pus cells in the exudate. However, as this is a mucous membrane, the initial vasodilatation means an increase in the production of mucus from the mucous glands. The pus

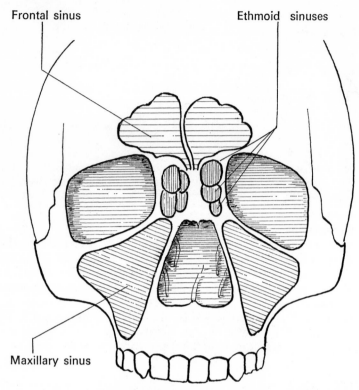

Frontal sinus

Ethmoid sinuses

Maxillary sinus

Fig. 31 Relationship of nasal sinuses (anterior view).

is not therefore pure pus, if one can have such a thing, but mucopus. The early production of fibrin seals off the natural ostium and, as a result, pus exerts pressure within the lumen of the sinus. If the pressure becomes too severe bone necrosis may occur, bacteraemia normally present may develop into septicaemia and pyaemia. Local thrombophlebitis may proliferate along venous channels to the meninges and meningitis and brain abscesses occur, leading to a fatal outcome.

CLINICAL PICTURE
The patient gives a history of having had a cold. After three or four days, at that point when the symptoms would have been expected to diminish, an exacerbation occurs. The nasal obstruction becomes worse and if there is drainage then the purulent nasal discharge increases. The sense of smell deteriorates and the patient feels a sense of fullness in the cheek on bending forwards. He feels toxic and wakes up in the morning with a headache which clears only when the increased congestion of the nose due to lying down has worn off.

On examination the patient has a watery-eyed heavy look. His tongue

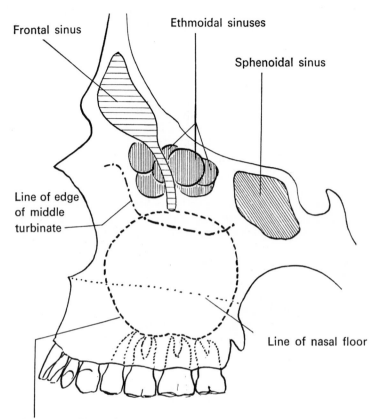

Frontal sinus

Ethmoidal sinuses

Sphenoidal sinus

Line of edge
of middle
turbinate

Line of nasal floor

Line of maxillary sinus

Fig. 32 Relationship of nasal sinuses. Note relation
of tooth roots to maxillary antrum.

is furred and he finds it difficult to keep his mouth closed. The temperature is raised. The nasal vestibule is red and excoriated. The nasal mucous membrane is very congested and it may be possible to see a trickle of thin pus from the middle meatus streaming backwards over the inferior turbinate and down into the post-nasal space. Pressure over the cheek below the eye may cause pain. This picture should suggest the diagnosis of acute sinusitis to the doctor. The diagnosis may be confirmed by investigations. These are:

(i) Culture of a nasal swab.

(ii) Radiology of the paranasal sinuses.

(iii) Total white cell count and blood sedimentation rate.

TREATMENT

General treatment
1 Rest
The patient with acute sinusitis who is both febrile and toxic should be nursed in bed. Every effort should be made to keep the room at an even temperature and humidity. This rests the nose as much as possible because it means that constant changes in the blood supply are not needed to warm and moisten the inspired air.

2 Hygiene
The patient should be well supplied with paper tissues for blowing the nose. If tissues are provided, then a container with a lid should also be provided for used tissues. Attention should also be paid to the mouth which tends to become very dry. The teeth should be brushed after every meal.

3 Diet
No special diet is called for. Plenty of fluids should be provided to keep the mouth well lubricated and to help to overcome the toxicity. If the nasal obstruction is severe the patient will find it more comfortable to drink with a drinking straw.

4 Drugs
Drugs used in the treatment of acute sinusitis are of two kinds. Symptomatic relief is obtained with salicylates or Paracetamol. Specific treatment is provided by antibiotics. Intramuscular penicillin is probably the safest and most effective treatment. A large dose of crystalline penicillin should be administered immediately AFTER the nasal swab has been taken and sent for culture and should be repeated every six hours for the first forty-eight hours. The patient can then be treated with a long-acting penicillin. If culture of the nasal swab shows that the organism is resistant to penicillin then the antibiotic should be chosen from the sensitivity test results. The antibiotic should not be stopped until at least forty-eight hours after all acute symptoms have subsided.

Local treatment—special measures

1 Inhalations
Inhalations are helpful in the adult patient because they save the nasal mucosa from work by providing air to breathe which is already warmed and moistened. They should never be ordered for small children because of the danger of scalding.

2 *Proof puncture and wash-out*

If the treatment outlined above does not bring about a rapid relief of symptoms and resolution of disease, there may be either poor drainage of the antrum or a resistant organism which has not been cultured from the nasal swab. Further information about these two points is obtained by a proof puncture and wash-out. A trocar and cannula are inserted through the naso-antral wall via the inferior meatus, under local anaesthesia. Sterile saline is introduced into the antrum and the contents of the antrum withdrawn into a syringe. If the drainage ostium is blocked then the extraction of the pus may prove to be very difficult. Any pus obtained should be sent for culture. If two or three wash-outs do not clear the infection it may be necessary to make an intranasal antrostomy (see chronic sinusitis, page 79).

ACUTE SINUSITIS OF INDIVIDUAL SINUSES

The maxillary sinuses are the ones most commonly affected by acute sinusitis and the above remarks apply particularly to disease of these sinuses. The other sinuses may be involved individually, however, as follows:

Ethmoiditis

In any attack of acute sinusitis the ethmoid sinuses are involved. The characteristic symptom is pain between and behind the eyes and severe nasal obstruction leading to a loss of the sense of smell. In the child there may be redness and oedema of the skin over the nasal bones and the medial side of the eye and cheek. Purulent epiphora may occur. The middle turbinate is covered with a fiercely congested mucous membrane and may be covered with thin mucopus. Ethmoidal sinusitis usually responds rapidly to the treatment which has been discussed above.

Frontal sinusitis

This may follow swimming or flying when the patient has a cold. It is usually unilateral. Severe headache over the eye is present in the morning on waking. The headache increases until the mid-morning, after which it tends to disappear in the late afternoon. Gentle pressure on the floor of the sinuses beside the nose may cause quite severe pain. There may be very little swelling of the mucous membrane of the nose to be seen. If the sinus is draining then mucopus is seen at the anterior end of the middle meatus. If no pus is seen it is of value to try the effect of a pledget of wool soaked in 1 : 1000 adrenaline hydrochloride solution. It may now be possible to see the drainage of pus and in this way too, pain may be relieved by relief of tension within the sinus cavity. If drainage cannot be promoted in this way it may be hindered by a poorly draining maxillary antrum. Antral wash-out may therefore be tried. Other measures which are sometimes helpful, before an actual attack on the sinus is considered, include amputation of the anterior end of the middle turbinate and submucous resection of the septum, if a septal spur is projecting into the middle meatus on the affected side.

However, it is imperative that the frontal sinus cavity should be emptied of pus if complications are to be avoided. Thus, if the measures outlined above fail, the floor of the frontal sinus will have to be trephined and a small drainage tube introduced.

Sphenoiditis
This condition may be more common than is usually stated. This is because it is extremely difficult to diagnose. It arises commonly in association with an acute ethmoiditis.

Clinical picture
The characteristic pain of an acute sphenoiditis is in the centre of the head. It radiates to the temporal regions and may on occasion be mistaken for earache. Very occasionally the pain is felt behind the eye. The patient may complain too of a purulent post-nasal discharge. He does not usually experience nasal obstruction. Very little may be seen on examination of the nose through the anterior nares. Pus may be seen on posterior rhinoscopy high up in the posterior choanae.

Sphenoidal sinusitis may respond to the treatment outlined above. However, if the symptoms persist it can be confirmed and relieved by washing out the sinus with a special sphenoidal sinus cannula.

Maxillary sinusitis of dental origin
Every now and then acute maxillary sinusitis follows dental sepsis or treatment. This is because the roots of the molar teeth in the upper jaw lie close to the floor of the maxillary antrum and may even protrude into it.

Clinical picture
The patient will give a history of toothache or of treatment for dental caries. Tenderness and swelling of the alveolar margin and of the lower part of the cheek may be seen. A characteristic feature of sinusitis of dental origin is the extremely foul-smelling nasal discharge. The causative organisms are not the usual streptococci, staphylococci and pneumococci. There is usually a profuse foul-smelling discharge to be seen in the nasal cavities.

Treatment
The conservative treatment given above should be pursued for three to four days. However, a broad spectrum antibiotic will be required to combat the infection. After three to four days the antrum should be washed out. This can be repeated if necessary. If the symptoms persist, drainage can be provided either by an intranasal antrostomy or the

antrum can be explored through the canine fossa and counter drainage into the nose established.

COMPLICATIONS OF ACUTE SINUSITIS

By definition, complication means that the disease is no longer confined to the organ affected and that other areas of the body have become involved. Classically, inflammations are said to spread by contiguity of tissue, by thrombophlebitis and by embolism. Sinusitis may spread in any or all of these three ways. The sinuses lie close to the brain and its coverings and to the orbit and its contents. Spread of acute infection from the sinuses can be dramatic and unless the complication is brought under control rapidly, can be fatal.

Spread to orbit

This usually results from a direct spread from the ethmoidal and frontal sinuses as a result of a destruction of the party wall between the sinus concerned and the orbit. It can, however, result from thrombophlebitis spreading from any of the sinuses.

Clinical picture

The patient gives a history of a preceding upper respiratory infection which has not cleared. A sudden increase in pain and toxaemia is associated with the development of an acute oedema of the eyelids, chemosis and diplopia. The eye may be displaced forwards or backwards by the swelling but is always displaced laterally. Usually by the time the patient is seen, pus has formed beneath the bone and the orbital periosteum. Unless the pus is drained rapidly, there is a danger of retrograde spread to the cavernous sinus and if this occurs, blindness may result from pressure on and around the optic nerve.

Treatment

This condition requires treatment as a matter of urgency if the eye is to be saved and further complications avoided.

A. The orbit should be drained if possible without entering the periorbital fat. Elevation of the orbital periosteum usually leads to an escape of pus which should be sent for culture and sensitivity.

B. Reinforcement of antibiotic therapy in order to prevent any extension of the disease. If antibiotics are already being administered, then it may be necessary to change the drug or to combine it with another antibiotic or sulphonamide preparation.

C. Drainage of the sinus from which the inflammation spread. This may necessitate the drainage of the antrum or the frontal sinus. Inflammation in the ethmoid sinuses will usually resolve if there is effective drainage of the antrum. None of these procedures should be carried out unless the patient has had time to build up an adequate concentration of antibiotic in the bloodstream.

Osteomyelitis of frontal bone

This is usually a disease of children and young adults. The majority of cases occur in boys and the causative organism is usually the staphylococcus pyogenes aureus or the anaerobic streptococcus. Since the frontal sinus does not appear until the sixth or seventh year, osteomyelitis of the frontal bone as an extension of frontal sinusitis is not seen until about the seventh or eighth year. However, it may follow trauma at an earlier age. There is often a history of trauma in the development of this condition. A blow on the head while playing football or diving into the water 'feet first' without pinching the nostrils can lead to damage to the mucosa of the sinuses. Most cases appear to be blood borne by a retrograde thrombophlebitis.

Clinical picture

Patients with this condition are very toxic and are frequently drowsy. It is difficult to obtain a clear history as to the onset as the malaise may have begun several weeks before the patient seeks advice. The disease tends to follow a cyclic course with exacerbations and remissions. There may be oedema of the upper eyelid and in almost all cases there will be a puffy swelling over the frontal bone (Pott's Puffy tumour). This swelling may be oedema or it may contain pus. However, it is important to bear in mind that in many cases there will be a corresponding swelling on the inner surface of the frontal bone. If the disease is untreated it extends upwards and backwards towards the vertex. Fistulae and sequestration of bone may take place. If the treatment is ineffective, then death may result from the development of intracranial suppuration. The diagnosis is established by the demonstration of a 'moth-eaten' appearance of the frontal bone on X-ray and by blood culture of the causative organism. It is important to set up both aerobic and anaerobic cultures at the time the patient is first seen because a significant percentage of these patients suffer from anaerobic infections. The progress of the disease is assessed by regular blood sedimentation rate estimations.

Treatment

When the patient is first admitted to hospital he should be treated with high dosage of crystalline penicillin given intramuscularly every six hours. If the blood culture shows that the staphylococcus is penicillin-resistant the treatment should be changed to fucidic acid or to an antibiotic which is appropriate to the organism's sensitivity. It is not possible to be dogmatic about the length of the course of antibiotic treatment. It should, however, be continued until all symptoms and signs have disappeared, and the blood sedimentation rate has become normal. Abscesses should be drained as they form and sequestra removed as required.

Osteomyelitis of maxilla

This is a rare complication of acute suppurative sinusitis. The reason for its inclusion in the list of complications is that it is frequently mistaken for sinusitis in infants and it is important that the diagnosis should be made early and the treatment begun if deformity is to be avoided and teeth saved.

Osteomyelitis of the maxilla usually follows a dental infection. In infants a buccal infection spreads to the dental sac and by a process of retrograde thrombophlebitis leads to necrosis of the upper jaw.

Clinical picture

The patient is usually an infant or young child. He presents with swelling of the cheek extending to the eye. There may be purulent epiphora and purulent nasal discharge. The alveolus is grossly swollen and this swelling extends to the mucous membrane of the hard palate reaching the midline. The child is acutely ill. If untreated, fistulae appear in the mouth and in due course sequestra are discharged through these fistulae.

Treatment

The condition usually responds rapidly to massive doses of intramuscular crystalline penicillin combined with the free drainage of any abscesses which may form. After the acute phase is over the antrum should be washed out in order to make sure that it contains no pus and that there is free drainage.

Intracranial complications

Infection may spread to the brain and its coverings by any of the three classical routes. However, it usually arises as a result of retrograde thrombophlebitis. There are well-established anatomical pathways through which the intracranial venous system may be involved. Thus, the cavernous sinus communicates directly with the sphenoids and via the pterygoid plexus with the maxillary antrum. In addition the diploetic veins in the frontal bone communicate with the superior sagittal sinus. Thrombophlebitis extending along any of these channels can lead to the development of any or all of the following complications:

1 Extra-dural abscess.
2 Sub-dural abscess.
3 Pachymeningitis.
4 Leptomeningitis.
5 Encephalitis.
6 Brain abscess.
7 Sagittal sinus thrombosis (otitic hydrocephalus).

For a full account of the clinical features of these conditions the reader should consult a textbook of neurology. For this book it must suffice to indicate the symptoms and signs which should suggest that such a complication has occurred.

Symptoms

1 Drowsiness alternating with normality.
2 Headache.
3 Fits.
4 Vomiting.
5 Weakness of the limbs.
6 Character changes.

Signs

1 Slowing pulse.
2 Difficulty in rousing.
3 Papilloedema.
4 Weakness of the limbs.
5 Swinging temperature.
6 Neck stiffness.
7 Positive Kernig's sign.
8 Inco-ordination and dysdiadochokinesia.
9 Loss of joint sensation.
10 Nystagmus.

The occurrence of any of the foregoing symptoms and signs should prompt further investigations, such as a plain X-ray of the skull to see whether there is any movement of the pineal body away from the midline, blood culture to isolate the causative organism and lumbar puncture providing that there is no evidence of grossly raised intracranial pressure which could produce pressure 'coning'.

The treatment of intracranial complications of adult sinus disease is based upon the use of the appropriate antibiotic combined with the drainage of any abscess which may form.

Chapter Fourteen
Chronic sinusitis

DEFINITION
A chronic inflammatory process affecting the mucosa and bony walls of the paranasal sinuses.

AETIOLOGY
Much has been written about the aetiology of chronic sinusitis. It is extremely difficult to prove any of the theories which seek to explain how the condition develops. There are in all probability many factors which lead to the development of the condition. Some of these are classified below.

Inadequate pneumatisation of sinuses
The diffuse inflammations of the upper respiratory tract which play such an important part in the development of immunity in the child have long been recognised. Attacks of inflammation follow each other in rapid succession and the interval between attacks may be so short that resolution is incomplete. The processes of inflammation and repair go 'hand in hand' and the resulting scar tissue formation narrows the ostium of the maxillary sinus and thus leads to inefficient aeration.

Inadequate diet
In the earlier years of this century, poverty frequently resulted in an inadequate diet. The child received too little food and that which was available was all too often unsuitable. As social conditions have improved nearly all children can expect to have an adequate diet but, due either to 'faddiness' or parental indifference, not all children have a suitable diet. Carbohydrates and milk are taken and proteins and vitamin foods are rejected and this can have a deleterious effect upon the respiratory mucosa.

Atopic reactions
The increasing complexity of man's way of life leads to an increase in hypersensitivity diseases. Hypersensitivity of the nasal mucous membrane leads to swelling and poor aeration of the sinuses.

Dirty environment

A dirty environment due to atmospheric pollution and 'self-inflicted' wounds in the form of alcohol and tobacco all lead to chronic congestion of the upper respiratory mucosa.

Dental sepsis

Chronic sinusitis is frequently associated with dental sepsis, but it is not always easy to decide which came first.

PATHOLOGY

There are three main categories of chronic sinusitis:

    (i) Sinusitis associated with simple inflammatory hyperplasia.
    (ii) Sinusitis as part of a generalised respiratory allergy.
    (iii) Either of the preceding types with infection superimposed.

Type (i) begins in early childhood. Recurrent bouts of infection occur. Remissions become shorter and shorter. The immune response becomes overwhelmed and resolution is never complete. The effect of this on the mucosa is a thickened basement membrane and dense lymphocytic infiltration. Sub-epithelial fibrosis leads to reduction in glandular tissue through ischaemia, and this may become so severe that actual ulceration of the mucosa may occur. At a later stage the periosteum becomes affected and hyperaemia extends to the bone, leading at first to osteoporosis and later to sclerosis.

Type (ii) is seen in those patients who have one of two types of allergy. The first is a generalised allergic diathesis presenting in early life with asthma, eczema, conjunctivitis and rhinitis and leading to seasonal rhinitis (hay fever) in middle childhood. In the second type there may be no symptom nor sign of allergy until eight or nine years of age after which a gradual 'waterlogging' of the mucosa leads to increasing nasal stuffiness and discharge. Polypi may be pulled down into the nasal cavity as a result of the pull of gravity on a waterlogged mucous membrane.

Once either of the two pathological states described becomes established, the condition is irreversible and such a patient cannot be cured. However, that does not mean that he cannot be helped by intelligent management.

SYMPTOMS AND SIGNS

In a disease where the onset is insidious the history tends to be vague and the patient presents with general complaints such as malaise, discomfort in the nose, 'catarrh'. It may be necessary to ask leading questions to discover whether the patient has:

    Nasal obstruction.
    Nasal discharge.
    Focal headache.
    Poor sense of smell and taste.

On clinical examination the mucous membrane is of a dull red colour and the nasal cavities may be seen to contain many dried crusts due to the excessive drying effect of the inspired air on the under-produced nasal mucus. The post-nasal space is inflamed and the lateral pharyngeal bands hypertrophic. The tongue is furred. Sinus X-rays commonly show thickening of the lining mucosa. They may, however, also show evidence of osteitis or osteosclerosis. Culture of a nasal swab will reveal a wide variety of organisms which may change from time to time. Most of these are saprophytic organisms or low-grade pathogens.

PROGNOSIS AND TREATMENT

The treatment of chronic sinusitis is palliative rather than curative. This is because, long before the patient seeks advice, irreversible changes have taken place within the lining of the nose and sinuses. These changes may have resulted in incomplete development of the sinuses and facial skeleton and naturally nothing can remedy such a disability. If the patient is not treated he will experience a great deal of minor ill health throughout his life. From time to time there will be acute exacerbations of the inflammation and there is always a possibility of the disease spreading beyond the confines of the sinuses. There is no line of demarcation in the respiratory tract between the 'upper' and the 'lower' portions and many patients who have chronic sinusitis also develop chest symptoms.

The palliative treatment which can be offered to the patient with chronic sinusitis will be discussed under:

(a) Conservative treatment.
(b) Radical treatment.

(a) Conservative treatment

Such measures are applied to the upper respiratory tract as a whole. The advice which is offered can, if followed, bring about a great improvement in the patient's general health and may delay or even make unnecessary any surgical procedure. There are two factors which need attention:

(i) The local nasal symptoms.
(ii) The demoralising effect which these symptoms have on the patient.

Such patients often lose regular patterns of life and behaviour and become weighed down by the burden of never feeling well and never being entirely free from nasal discomfort.

The first objective in conservative treatment is therefore to bring about a return to 'regular habits'. This means that adequate rest, adequate diet and adequate exercise must be ordered. At the beginning of treatment a dental examination should be carried out and any caries found put right. The three universal or almost universal aggravating factors, dust, alcohol and tobacco, must be considered and wherever possible adjustments made. A holiday in a clean dry climate will always bring some temporary improvement and can, if timed strategically, give impetus to other measures and give the patient confidence in the efficacy of the treatment.

Periods of acute secondary infection of the chronic inflammatory process are inevitable. They should be treated vigorously, if necessary by the exhibition of antibiotics in full courses. The inexperienced doctor should however beware. There is a great tendency for patients debilitated by much minor ill health to take their medicine only until such time as they feel better and then to preserve 'what is left' against the next recrudescence so that they have something in hand and will not have to trouble the doctor. The doctor should therefore make it his business to see that the antibiotic prescribed is taken in the right dosage and at the right time. The patient will also get relief at times from the use of steam inhalations.

These are measures which, if deployed with judgement, can tide a patient over successfully without recourse to surgery for many years. There is one form of conservative treatment which should be mentioned only so that it may be condemned. NO PATIENT WITH CHRONIC NASAL OBSTRUCTION SHOULD BE ALLOWED TO USE VASOCONSTRICTOR DROPS OR SPRAYS. These preparations produce ONLY a temporary improvement in the airway. As the effect wears off a reactionary swelling of the mucosa takes place and soon the actual chemicals in the spray produce an irritative response within the lining of the nose and the disease process is aggravated rather than alleviated.

(b) Radical treatment

In the past the surgical treatment of chronic sinusitis has not enjoyed a good reputation. This is because on the whole the surgeon sought to cure the incurable and failed to explain the objectives to be achieved by surgery to his patient. Very radical treatment such as stripping of the lining mucosa and obliteration procedures should be reserved for severe and intractable cases. Much, however, can be done by minor surgical procedures designed to improve drainage and the airway. These will be considered for individual sinuses.

Maxillary sinus

Long-term narrowing of the ostium of the maxillary sinus can lead to a small antrum with a mucosa which is non-functional. The ciliary mechanisms fail and the sinus cavity becomes filled with viscid mucus. In such an environment low-grade pathogens flourish and one may recover *Haemophilus influenzae* and on occasion *B. proteus* and *E. coli*. When this condition is confirmed by radiology and by proof puncture, great relief can be obtained by making an intranasal antrostomy. This

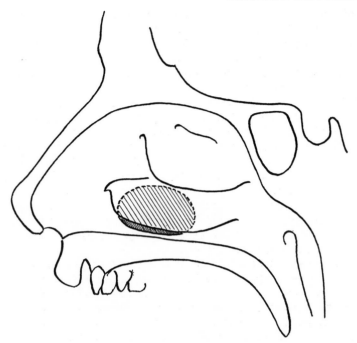

Fig. 33 Site of intranasal antrostomy.

is an artificial opening into the antrum made low down in the inferior meatus. The antrum then empties itself by the action of gravity. If the lining of the antrum is polypoidal and in addition the infection has spread deep to the mucosa involving the bony sinus wall it may be necessary to remove the lining and to provide dependent drainage. This operation (Caldwell–Luc) is carried out through the canine fossa. It is required only rarely but can give considerable relief.

Frontal sinus

Operations on the frontal sinus may be called for when there is intractable pain in the region of the frontal sinus due to osteitis or when the disease process spreads beyond the frontal sinus and complications develop. The surgeon may decide

    1 to refashion the sinus and the fronto-nasal duct, or
    2 to excise the sinus and to obliterate the space left behind.

Neither procedure enjoys universal commendation. There are formidable anatomical difficulties to be overcome and unfortunately the disease tends to recur so that further operations may be called for.

Ethmoidal sinus

Chronic inflammation of the ethmoidal sinus usually presents with nasal

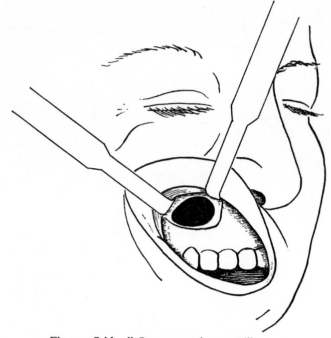

Fig. 34 Caldwell–Luc approach to maxillary antrum.

polypi which are causing nasal obstruction and which are associated with a secondary infection. The patient is troubled by nasal obstruction and anosmia, nasal discharge and headache. The health is generally poor and may be worsened when lower respiratory symptoms supervene.

The ethmoid sinus may be approached in three ways.

1 Intranasally

This route is the approach of choice when the disease is limited to the ethmoid sinus. All diseased bone and lining is punched away under direct vision leaving the shell of the middle turbinate behind. A detailed knowledge of the anatomy of the ethmoid is required before this can be accomplished safely.

2 Frontal ethmoidal approach

Here the frontals and ethmoids are exposed together through an incision medial to the inner canthus of the eye. It is reserved for infections of both the frontal and the ethmoidal sinuses occurring together.

3 Transantral ethmoidal approach

This operation, carried out through the canine fossa, is reserved for disease affecting the antra and ethmoid sinuses together.

FRONTAL MUCOCELE

This condition must be mentioned as a separate entity because of its unusual clinical presentation.

Pathology

Following obstruction to the drainage of the fronto-nasal duct by chronic inflammation, the lumen of the sinus becomes filled with an encysted collection of mucus. The mucus tends to increase in quantity gradually and the sinus wall and floor move away due to the pressure of the fluid. In due course the contour of the sinus is changed and the wall greatly thinned. If the condition is still untreated, then super-added secondary infection may lead to the development of a pyocele.

Clinical picture

The patient who is usually of middle age presents with a swelling above and medial to the orbit. If the swelling, which is usually painless, is large enough there will be some disturbance of vision due to pressure on the globe. The swelling should be palpated gently because if the bony floor of the sinus is greatly thinned 'egg-shell crackling' may be elicited. This is due to comminution of the sinus floor. The diagnosis is confirmed radiologically.

Treatment

Frontal mucoceles have to be removed through an external incision. All unhealthy mucosa is excised and adequate drainage of the sinus into the nose is established.

Chapter Fifteen
Tumours of the nose, sinuses and nasopharynx

These tumours are not common. Their presenting symptoms, however, do not always indicate the serious nature of the underlying disease and the most important point is for the practitioner to be aware of the early symptoms of these tumours.

BENIGN TUMOURS

Nose and sinuses
Benign tumours of the nose and sinuses are uncommon, the commonest being the squamous papilloma (Ringertz tumour). This tumour usually causes nasal obstruction. It should be removed surgically but tends to recur and rarely takes on malignant characteristics.

The other benign tumour of importance, although it is uncommon, is the osteoma. This affects the frontal sinus most often; it may be symptomless but if it occludes the fronto-nasal duct it will give rise to recurrent attacks of acute frontal sinusitis. It may also expand downwards into the orbit or backwards to erode the meninges. In the latter case recurrent attacks of meningitis occur. If these tumours are causing symptoms they should be removed by an external approach.

Nasopharynx
Benign tumours of the nasopharynx are uncommon, the most important being the nasopharyngeal angio-fibroma. This tumour occurs only in boys about the age of puberty. It is a large fleshy tumour which usually presents with epistaxis and if untreated expands to invade the orbit and skull. It should, therefore, be removed surgically but this is hazardous because of the torrential haemorrhage which usually follows manipulation of these tumours. Cryosurgery, however, offers the hope that these uncommon but difficult tumours may in the near future be dealt with more easily.

MALIGNANT TUMOURS OF THE SINUSES
Malignant tumours of the sphenoid and frontal sinuses are very rare. Tumours of the ethmoid sinuses cannot be distinguished from tumours

of the lateral wall of the nose and will be considered with these latter tumours. The only tumours to be considered here, therefore, are tumours of the maxillary antrum.

Pathology

A malignant tumour of the antrum usually involves the entire cavity and it is generally impossible to say where the tumour originated. The tumour does not usually present until it has spread beyond one of the walls of the antrum. Metastases to lymph nodes in the neck are uncommon and do not usually occur until the tumour has invaded a rich lymphatic area such as the cheek or the hard palate. Distant metastases are uncommon.

Although the antrum is lined by columnar epithelium, most malignant tumours are squamous carcinomata; this indicates that the tumour is preceded by squamous metaplasia. Adenocarcinomata do occasionally occur at this site, however; they are usually primary but may be secondary from a hypernephroma or seminoma.

Presenting symptoms

A carcinoma of the antrum may present in the following ways:

Nasal symptoms

If the tumour spreads through the medial wall of the antrum into the nose, there will be *unilateral* nasal obstruction and a blood-stained nasal discharge. Pain in the face may also occur.

Facial symptoms

Swelling of the face is a fairly common, but late symptom. Pain and numbness may also occur.

Eye symptoms

The tumour may spread through the roof of the antrum, invade the orbit and produce either proptosis or lateral displacement of the eyeball. In this event the patient will usually present to the ophthalmologist. Uncommonly a patient may also present to the eye department because of unilateral epiphora caused by invasion of the naso-lacrimal duct.

Dental symptoms

A tumour may invade downwards on to the hard palate. The patient will then present to a dentist with pain or loosening of the teeth, or with a swelling or ulceration of the hard palate.

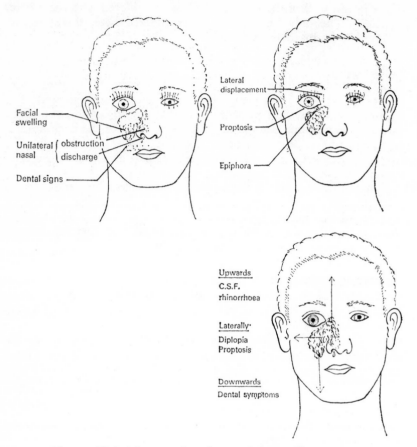

Facial swelling

Unilateral nasal { obstruction discharge

Dental signs

Lateral displacement

Proptosis

Epiphora

Upwards
C.S.F. rhinorrhoea

Laterally·
Diplopia
Proptosis

Downwards
Dental symptoms

Fig. 35 Clinical features of carcinoma of the maxillary antrum.

Investigations

Radiology
Radiology of the sinuses shows the involved antrum to be opaque on X-ray, with destruction of one of its bony walls.

Biopsy
Although a specimen of tumour for biopsy can often be obtained from the nose, the antrum should always be explored through a Caldwell–Luc approach, through its anterior wall. This serves two purposes: a specimen can be obtained for biopsy and an antrostomy into the nose is created. The latter allows drainage when the patient is irradiated.

Treatment
The accepted treatment policy for these tumours is a combination of radiotherapy and surgery. The antrum is first irradiated with a dose of 5500 rads. This causes much sloughing and discharge from the antral cavity; hence the importance of providing drainage before radiotherapy begins. Two months after the therapy is finished a palatal fenestration is carried out. In this operation, the hard palate, any involved part of the alveolar ridge and the medial wall of the antrum are removed to create a large cavity. The defect in the hard palate is subsequently closed by a dental plate so that the patient can speak and eat normally. The purpose of this operation is to remove any residual cancer and to make it easy to see into the cavity, which should be inspected every month for the first two years and every three months thereafter. A recurrence can thus be seen early and treated by total maxillectomy. If an enlarged node in the neck appears a block dissection should be done. This policy produces a five-year cure rate of 40%.

MALIGNANT NASAL TUMOURS
Malignant tumours of the nose are uncommon; they almost always affect the lateral wall and are indistinguishable from tumours of the ethmoid sinuses.

Pathology
These tumours are usually squamous carcinomata. They produce oedema of the nasal mucosa because of interference with its lymphatic or venous drainage; a polypoid mass then forms. Invasion upwards into the anterior cranial fossa and laterally into the orbit occurs. Lymph nodes metastases in the neck are uncommon, as are distant metastases.

Clinical features
These tumours usually present with nasal signs; there is unilateral nasal obstruction and a blood stained nasal discharge. Because of orbital invasion they may present with diplopia or proptosis. Rarely invasion of the anterior cranial fossa causes a cerebrospinal rhinorrhoea.

Treatment
Radiotherapy is the first line of treatment. The patient should be seen at monthly intervals thereafter and a recurrence treated by excision of the lateral wall of the nasal cavity through a lateral rhinotomy.

MALIGNANT TUMOURS OF THE NASOPHARYNX
Tumours of the nasopharynx are uncommon in Great Britain, but for some unknown reason they are one of the commonest tumours in the Far East.

Pathology

Tumours of the nasopharynx arise from the lateral wall or the roof and are usually infiltrating rather than papilliferous.

The nasopharynx is a rich lymphatic area so that many of these patients have an enlarged node in the neck when first seen. Also reticuloses are often seen at this site.

Histology

A great variety of tumours occur in the nasopharynx. A squamous carcinoma is the commonest but reticuloses are frequently seen, particularly lymphosarcoma and reticulum cell sarcoma.

Presenting symptoms

Tumours of the nasopharynx present in several different ways, none of which obviously suggests that such a lesion is present because the primary tumour in the nasopharynx does not itself cause symptoms. These tumours then present to several different specialists because they do not cause symptoms until spread has occurred.

Neck mass

An enlarged gland in the neck occurs in three patients out of four with a nasopharyngeal cancer; it is the presenting symptom in about half of them. As the tumour in the nasopharynx causes no symptoms the patient's only complaint is of the neck mass. In such a patient the nasopharynx must be examined and any suspicious area biopsied before a biopsy of the neck mass is carried out.

Unilateral deafness

A tumour of the lateral wall of the nasopharynx invades the medial end of the Eustachian tube which then becomes obstructed. This leads to a serous otitis media causing a unilateral conductive deafness.

Cranial nerve paralyses

A nasopharyngeal tumour may invade the base of the skull in two directions. Invasion upwards through the foramen lacerum results in a lesion of the nerves in the lateral wall of the cavernous sinus—the third, fourth and sixth cranial nerves and the ophthalmic division of the fifth cranial nerve. There may thus be an ophthalmoplegia or pain in the face.

Invasion laterally and backwards along the base of the skull destroys the nerves passing through the jugular foramen—the ninth, tenth and eleventh cranial nerves causing a motor or sensory paralysis of the pharynx or larynx.

Nasal symptoms

The patient may present with epistaxis or with nasal obstruction if the tumour is large.

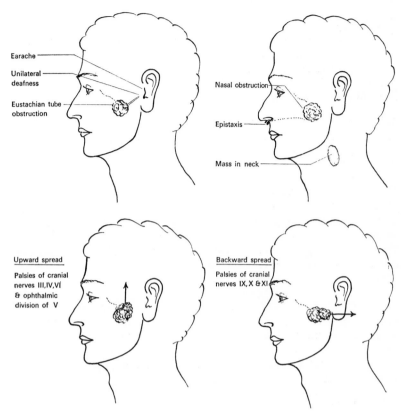

Fig. 36 Presenting symptoms of carcinoma of nasopharynx.

Investigations

The nasopharynx is inspected under general anaesthetic and a specimen obtained for biopsy.

A radiograph of the base of the skull is taken to delineate any bony destruction.

Treatment

Radiotherapy is the only possible treatment for a nasopharyngeal cancer whatever its histological type. An enlarged gland in the neck is treated by a block dissection provided the primary tumour has healed.

Prognosis

The outlook in this disease is poor; one patient in five will survive five years.

Chapter Sixteen
Symptoms and signs of throat disease

SYMPTOMS

Sore throat, hoarseness and dysphagia are the common symptoms of throat disease. All of these symptoms can occur in children or young adults, usually lasting for a few days only and accompanied by systemic symptoms such as fever; in such patients the cause is infection. If these symptoms occur in a patient over the age of forty-five, however, particularly if they are not accompanied by systemic symptoms and if they persist, they are almost certainly caused by a carcinoma of the upper respiratory or digestive tracts.

Sore throat

A patient may complain of a sore throat lasting a few days or he may complain of a persistent sore throat over many weeks or months. It is important, therefore, to ask a patient complaining of sore throats whether they last for a few days only and are accompanied by systemic symptoms such as a fever, or whether the sore throat is persistent and usually unaccompanied by other symptoms. A sore throat lasting a few days only is obviously caused by acute infection, either viral or bacterial, and is commonly seen in children and young adults.

A persistent sore throat, occurring in young and middle-aged adults, is usually due to chronic pharyngitis and/or laryngitis; often there are no other symptoms, no systemic upset and no dysphagia. Such a sore throat is often worse in the morning due to mouth-breathing at night.

The pharynx and larynx lie at the junction of the upper and lower respiratory tracts and may therefore be subject to irritation by disease of either of these tracts. Thus, if a patient suffers from nasal obstruction, caused by a deflected nasal septum, nasal polypi, vasomotor rhinitis or sinusitis, he will breathe through his mouth and irritate his larynx and pharynx with cold dry air. In many of these diseases there may also be a purulent post-nasal discharge which also irritates the pharynx and larynx.

In addition the pharynx and larynx may be irritated by diseases of the lower respiratory tract, particularly in a patient with chronic bronchitis associated with purulent sputum. Also they may be subject to local irritation by smoking, drinking and abuse of the voice, and by secondary infection due to carious teeth. It is obviously important, therefore, in a patient with a persistent sore throat to ask about nasal discharge and obstruction and to ask about his general health, in particular his chest; these regions must also be examined in any patient with a persistent sore throat as also must the teeth.

Finally, it should be remembered that occasionally a persistent sore throat in a patient in the cancer age group may be the only presenting symptom of a pharyngeal or laryngeal tumour.

Hoarseness

Hoarseness may occur in short-lived attacks or may persist. A short, acute attack of hoarseness accompanied by a systemic upset is due to acute laryngitis, which is usually a part of a generalised upper respiratory infection. Persistent hoarseness, however, is caused either by chronic laryngitis, by a paralysis of a vocal cord or by a tumour of the larynx. Chronic laryngitis is usually secondary to the same forms of irritation as chronic pharyngitis described above.

Hoarseness due to a paralysis of the vocal cord is often secondary to a carcinoma of the bronchus and it is, therefore, important to enquire about symptoms of chest disease.

Finally, a tumour of the larynx usually causes hoarseness only and there are often no other symptoms until late in the disease. It is important, therefore, in any patient with persistent hoarseness and nc other symptoms to suspect a carcinoma of the larynx.

Any patient more than forty years old, who has been hoarse for more than two consecutive weeks, should be considered to be suffering from laryngeal cancer, until conclusively proven otherwise. It is, therefore, essential for his larynx to be examined with a laryngeal mirror. Should the doctor be inexperienced with this procedure, the patient should then be referred to hospital for the opinion of a laryngologist.

Dysphagia

Dysphagia may be caused by lesions either within the lumen of the oesophagus or within its wall or by pressure from outside the lumen.

A patient with an organic lesion of the oesophagus complains first of difficulty in swallowing solid foods. Later he is unable to swallow liquids and finally his own saliva. Occasionally the first complaint may be of difficulty in swallowing liquids; this is typically seen in achalasia of the oesophagus. In an organic obstruction of the oesophagus the patient can often localise the point at which food sticks. Pain on swallowing usually indicates a lesion in the pharynx, and this pain often radiates to one or both ears. Dysphagia also occurs in acute infections such as tonsillitis but in these patients obviously only lasts for a few days.

In practice any patient who has difficulty in swallowing SOLID food for more than two weeks should be assumed to have cancer of the pharynx or oesophagus until proven otherwise.

Long-standing oesophageal obstruction obviously affects the patient's general health so that there is loss of weight and energy. In addition there may be spill-over of food or saliva into the chest causing recurrent attacks of broncho-pneumonia.

Lump in the Throat (*Globus hystericus*)

Many patients complain of a lump in the throat, usually in the midline located just above the suprasternal notch; the symptom often improves with swallowing food. They are usually middle-aged women who have no difficulty whatsoever in swallowing solid food, have no other throat symptoms and have not lost weight. Examination in these patients reveals no abnormality and the condition may be due to spasm of the pharyngeal constrictor muscles, but some of these patients on investigation are found to have reflux oesophagitis.

EXAMINATION

The requirements for carrying out an adequate examination of the mouth are a light, and two spatulae. It is thus obvious that a source of light cannot be held in one of the examiner's hands but must come from an overhead light, preferably from a forehead lamp. The mouth should be examined systematically as follows.

The teeth and alveolar ridges should be examined; dental caries may lead to chronic pharyngitis and is often the cause of persistent sore throat.

The cheek should be held aside with a spatula and its mucosal lining examined. The most common abnormality is hyperkeratosis which presents an appearance of white patches. While examining the inner surface of the cheek, the opening of the parotid duct, opposite the second upper molar tooth, should be examined. The anterior two-thirds of the tongue should be examined and its mobility estimated by asking the patient to put out his tongue. The inferior surface, including the opening of the sub-mandibular duct, should also be examined. It is very important to inspect the sulcus lying between the lower alveolar margin and the tongue, and this can only be carried out with two spatulae to open up the sulcus. Tumours may occur at this site and if this examination is omitted they may be missed.

The palate is inspected and its mobility estimated by asking the patient to say 'ah'. The tonsils should be examined, and lastly, the visible area of the posterior pharyngeal wall should be inspected.

The mouth should also be palpated. Thus it may be possible to feel stones in the sub-mandibular gland or duct. If a tumour is found in the oral cavity it should be palpated to determine its extent.

The pharynx and larynx are now examined with a laryngeal mirror and a reflected light. The patient is asked to put out his tongue, which

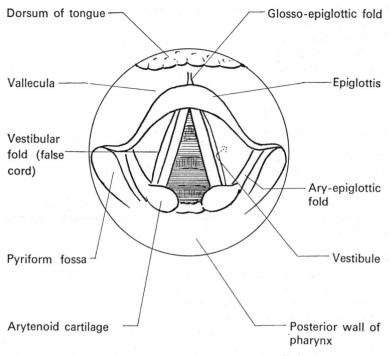

Fig. 37 The Larynx on mirror examination (indirect laryngoscopy).

is held gently with a gauze swab. A warm laryngeal mirror is then introduced gently but firmly, to lift up the soft palate. At this stage the upper part of the epiglottis, the base of the tongue and the posterior pharyngeal wall can be seen, but the larynx cannot be seen because it lies under the epiglottis and base of tongue. The larynx is brought into view by asking the patient to say 'ee'. This manoeuvre elevates the larynx and tilts the epiglottis forwards. The larynx and pharynx should then be examined systematically: both sides of the epiglottis, the ary-epiglottic folds, the false cords and the arytenoids, the pyriform fossa and the posterior pharyngeal wall are examined. The mobility of the vocal cords is assessed by asking the patient again to say 'ee' and to take a deep breath. Any inflammation, ulceration, mucosal irregularity or fixation of the larynx are noted.

Palpation of the neck
The lymph nodes of the neck are often enlarged in diseases of the pharynx, larynx and mouth so that no examination of the throat is complete without palpation of the neck.

The neck is palpated from behind and its regions examined in an orderly sequence starting at the posterior triangle, proceeding up the jugular chain and finishing with the anterior triangle. The tension of the sterno-mastoid muscle is relaxed by turning the patient's head to the same side so that it is easier to palpate any enlarged nodes in the jugular chain. If a lump is felt, its size, site, shape, consistency and fixation to adjacent tissues are noted; also whether it moves on swallowing.

INVESTIGATIONS

General Investigation
Diseases of the larynx and pharynx are often caused by disease elsewhere, particularly in other parts of the respiratory tract. Also any prolonged disorder of the larynx or pharynx often has a profound effect on the patient's general health; this should therefore be assessed before specialised investigations are carried out.

Chest X-ray
An X-ray of the chest should be taken for two reasons: disease of the larynx may be secondary to chest disease, and, conversely, diseases of the larynx may cause pulmonary disorders. Common examples of laryngeal diseases secondary to chest disease are a vocal cord paralysis caused by a bronchial carcinoma and chronic laryngitis secondary to chronic bronchitis with purulent sputum; though uncommon, laryngeal tuberculosis is always secondary to pulmonary tuberculosis. Pulmonary disease secondary to laryngeal disease may arise as follows: a carcinoma of the larynx or pharynx does not often produce generalised metastases but if it does the lungs are the commonest site to be affected. Also, long-standing disease of the larynx or pharynx, for example a pharyngeal pouch, is often associated with spill-over, causing pulmonary infection.

Sinus X-ray
An X-ray of the sinuses must also be taken; it may show an infection which could be the cause of a chronic laryngitis.

Bacteriology
A nasal swab, throat swab and specimen of sputum should always be cultured in any infection of the upper respiratory tract.

Haematology
A haemoglobin estimation and white cell count with a differential count will usually be needed in an infection of the larynx or pharynx. A Paul Bunnell test may also be required occasionally in a patient with pharyngeal ulceration.

In the older patient, particularly if a carcinoma is suspected, a more detailed estimation of the patient's general health is required. The blood urea, blood sugar, electrolytes and serum protein should therefore be estimated.

Syphilis of the larynx is now rarely seen, but a W.R. should be done if a tumour of the larynx is seen, because gummatous laryngitis and a carcinoma may co-exist and are clinically indistinguishable from each other.

The patient should be weighed, the figure to be compared with his usual weight and to act as a yardstick during any subsequent treatment.

Local investigation

In many cases, if the patient is only suffering from acute or chronic infection of the larynx or pharynx, a diagnosis can usually be arrived at by taking a history and carrying out a simple examination of the pharynx and larynx.

If the history suggests that the patient may be suffering from malignancy, or if there is any mucosal abnormality of the larynx or pharynx, investigations should be completed by radiology and by examination under anaesthetic; neither of these steps must be omitted.

Radiology

A barium swallow will usually show any organic lesion of the pharynx or oesophagus. Occasionally, however, a lesion may not be demonstrated; a normal report should be ignored if the patient has difficulty in swallowing food and an oesophagoscopy carried out.

The larynx can be demonstrated radiologically by tomography or by laryngography. The latter is a double contrast technique in which the larynx is outlined by a radio-opaque material. To obtain good films with this technique the larynx must first be anaesthetised.

Examination under anaesthetic

Finally the larynx, pharynx and oesophagus are examined under anaesthetic. This step enables inaccessible parts of the larynx and pharynx to be seen and mucosal irregularities to be biopsied. Oesophagoscopy must always be done in a patient who has dysphagia for food, even if a barium swallow is reported as normal.

The larynx is first examined with a laryngoscope. This allows the surgeon to examine the vallecula, both surfaces of the epiglottis, the false cords, the true cords and the sub-glottic area. Lastly an oesophagoscope is introduced, through which the pyriform fossa and the entire length of the oesophagus are examined. Ulceration, tumours, strictures and the presence of free fluid are looked for; a biopsy is taken from any suspected area of mucosa; if free fluid is present it is tested with blue litmus paper to ascertain if it is acid, indicating reflux oesophagitis.

Chapter Seventeen
Diseases of the tonsils and adenoid

LIFE HISTORY OF THE TONSILS AND ADENOIDS
Acute infections of the upper respiratory tract in children form a large part of the work of a general practitioner. There is also much controversy over the medical and surgical treatment of these diseases. Because both medical and surgical treatment are dictated by the physiological changes which take place in the growing child, it is essential first to consider the physiology of the tonsils and adenoids.

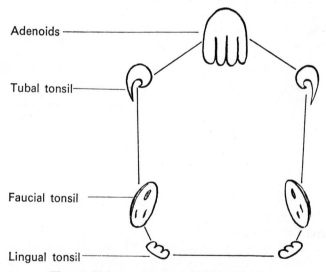

Adenoids

Tubal tonsil

Faucial tonsil

Lingual tonsil

Fig. 38 Main components of Waldeyer's ring.

The tonsils and adenoids form part of the ring of lymphoid tissue at the entrance to the respiratory and digestive tracts known as Waldeyer's ring. The other members of this ring are the lingual tonsils and the lymphoid tissue in the mouth of the Eustachian tube. This collection of tissue, at the entrance to the respiratory and digestive tracts, protects the child from inhaled and ingested infection. Like all other lymphoid tissue, the contents of Waldeyer's ring hypertrophy during childhood and atrophy after puberty. Also this collection of tissue functions as a unit so that during its active phase, removal of one part leads to hypertrophy of the remaining tissue.

The tonsils and adenoids are small at birth. During childhood they both undergo physiological hypertrophy, the adenoids at the age of three and the tonsils at five. Because the adenoids are large, mouth-breathing occurs, the tonsils are thus exposed to the inspired air and they also enlarge.

At the age of five the child goes to school and is exposed to infection from other children. This also causes the tonsils to enlarge.

After the age of five both structures shrink but the tonsils enlarge again at the age of ten. Both structures finally atrophy at puberty, the adenoids disappearing entirely and the tonsils becoming very small.

A diagrammatic growth curve is shown in Fig. 39.

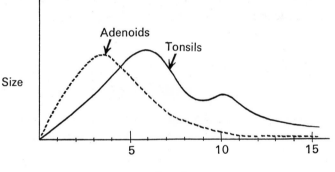

Fig. 39 Growth curves of tonsils and adenoids.

ACUTE TONSILLITIS AND TONSILLECTOMY

Tonsillitis in children
Acute tonsillitis occurs most often in children. In a child it differs from the disease in an adult and will therefore be discussed separately.

Pathology
Acute tonsillitis occurs most often about the age of five with a second peak at the age of ten. As can be seen from the accompanying figure, pathogenic bacteria can only be isolated in approximately half the cases, the remainder being due to viruses.

It is impossible by looking at the tonsils to know whether infection is due to bacteria or to viruses, and therefore inspection is of no help in deciding which patients should be treated by antibiotics.

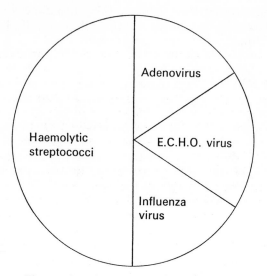

Fig. 40 Causal organisms of acute tonsillitis.

Clinical features

The child is obviously ill and feverish. A child who is too young to talk does not complain specifically about his throat, so that it is important to examine the upper respiratory tract of every child with an unexplained fever. The older child complains of a sore throat and has obvious difficulty in swallowing.

The tonsils are inflamed, swollen and covered by pus and exudate. The jugulo-digastric lymph nodes are enlarged and tender.

Differential diagnosis

A. *Infectious mononucleosis* may be indistinguishable clinically from acute tonsillitis and on occasion a differential white count and Paul Bunnell test will be required.

B. *Vincent's angina* causes widespread ulceration of the mouth but may occasionally be localised to the fauces. It can be readily distinguished from tonsillitis by a throat swab.

C. *Agranulocytosis* may present with ulceration of the mouth or pharynx. Ulceration and sloughing of the mucous membrane of the mouth, tongue and tonsils is widespread and the patient is obviously very ill. A white cell count provides the diagnosis.

Complications

A quinsy (q.v.) is the only common local complication of tonsillitis. Rheumatic fever and nephritis can follow a streptococcal tonsillitis, but these complications are not as frequent as they used to be.

Treatment

A. Throat swab
If practicable a throat swab should be taken for culture and sensitivity.

B. General measures
Until the result of a throat swab is known most patients can be made comfortable by aspirin. If a young child is ill enough he will stay in bed voluntarily, but if he will not, there is little point in insisting on this.

C. Antibiotic therapy
Most attacks of tonsillitis will resolve without antibiotic therapy which is not indicated anyway if the infection is caused by a virus. Antibiotics are therefore justifiable only in the following circumstances:

(a) Lack of response to the above general measures after two days with continuing high fever.

(b) Isolation of a haemolytic streptococcus from a throat swab.

Penicillin is still the best antibiotic, preferably administered intramuscularly, in a dose of 250 000 units six-hourly. In general practice this is rarely practicable and it is usual to give oral penicillin, for example phenoxymethyl penicillin (penicillin V) 125 mg six-hourly. It is important to impress on the child's parents that the medicine must be given regularly and for a full five days, otherwise rapidly recurring infection can be caused. About a quarter of haemolytic streptococci are no longer sensitive to the tetracycline group of drugs and these should not therefore be used.

TONSILLECTOMY
The indications for tonsillectomy have for a long time caused much controversy. Approximately 200 000 children a year in this country have their tonsils removed, many of whom probably derive no real benefit from the operation; certainly the few children who die of the operation do not.

The reason that controversy has arisen about the indications for tonsillectomy is that there are no objective signs on which to judge the issue. No convincing evidence has ever been produced to show which child should have its tonsils removed or whether the operation will do him any good. It is surprising that there is no proof available of the benefits of an operation which has been carried out millions of times.

Perhaps because the issue is always decided on subjective grounds, several interesting anomalies in the incidence of tonsillectomy have arisen.

Thus the Registrar-General's statistics show that infective respiratory diseases are commoner in the lower social classes and are commoner in the North-West of England than on the South Coast. The incidence of tonsillectomy ought therefore to be highest in the lower social classes living in the North-West of England. However, measurement of the incidence of tonsillectomy in representative samples, such as recruits to the Armed Forces, shows that tonsillectomy is most often carried out in children of the higher social classes, particularly those living in the South of England.

Since no evidence is available to indicate the place of this operation, common sense dictates that we remember that all children ultimately grow out of these diseases; a child should therefore only be subjected to an unpleasant and potentially dangerous operation if it suffers attacks of tonsillitis of such frequency and severity as to make the operation worth while. This can only be decided on the history. Examination of the mouth establishes one fact only—that the tonsils are present. No other information can be obtained by looking at the tonsils to help in deciding whether they should be removed.

In eliciting a history two points should be established:

Firstly, are the tonsils themselves the actual site of the infection? Tonsillitis is a self-limiting disease lasting about *five days* with *dysphagia* and a *fever*. If the recurrent attacks do not comply with such a picture the child is more likely to be suffering from chronic pharyngitis caused by infection of the nose or sinuses, dental sepsis or mouth breathing. The sore throat of chronic pharyngitis tends to be persistent, often worse in the morning and unaccompanied by dysphagia and pyrexia.

Secondly, are these attacks of tonsillitis causing sufficient disability to justify tonsillectomy? If a child often has severe attacks of acute tonsillitis he will lose a lot of school and because he cannot eat during the attacks will not gain weight and may even lose weight. These two factors—loss of school and loss of weight—are of great help in deciding that tonsillectomy is justified. If, however, the child has not lost very much school, is gaining weight and looks fit, he should be left alone to grow out of his troubles.

A child who has had a quinsy (q.v.) should also have his tonsils removed as he is in danger of having a further attack which may be complicated by spreading infection in the fascial planes of the neck. However, a quinsy is commoner in adults as a complication of tonsillitis.

To summarise, a child who has had frequent attacks of acute tonsillitis, say five or six times a year, who has lost a lot of time off school and who is not gaining weight, should have his tonsils removed. But a child who is fit and healthy, who loses little school, should be left alone.

Conditions under which the tonsils should not be removed

Acute upper respiratory infection
The tonsils should not be removed during or for three weeks after an acute attack of tonsillitis because of the danger of secondary haemorrhage.

Blood dyscrasias

If the bleeding or clotting time is prolonged, for example in haemo-philia or purpura, tonsillectomy is never justifiable.

Cleft palate

A cleft palate causes incompetence of the nasopharyngeal sphincter and even after repair may be inadequate and may not meet the posterior pharyngeal wall so that the child has unsatisfactory speech. In such a child the tonsils should only be removed if they are causing severe symptoms, and then only by an expert, as any scarring of the soft palate after operation leads to further incompetence of the nasopharyngeal sphincter.

Rheumatic fever and nephritis

Tonsillectomy was previously advised in these conditions to prevent recurrence. Most paediatricians and E.N.T. surgeons now feel that, as patients who have suffered from these two diseases are generally maintained on long-term prophylactic penicillin, there is little point in carrying out tonsillectomy. However, despite prophylactic antibiotics, occasionally a child continues to have attacks of streptococcal tonsillitis and to prevent a recurrence of the rheumatic fever or nephritis it is justifiable in such a child to carry out tonsillectomy. The operation must be carried out under penicillin cover.

Poliomyelitis

The tonsils and adenoids should not be removed during a poliomye-litis epidemic because of the increased risk of contracting the disease. There is also a greater risk of bulbar poliomyelitis developing in a patient who has recently had his tonsils removed.

Enlargement of tonsils

It will be noted that enlargement of the tonsils has not been given as an indication for their removal. Hypertrophy of the tonsils occurs nor-mally at certain periods in a child's life and it is reasonable to suppose that the cause of this lies in stimulation by infection. To remove the tonsils only because they are large is therefore not only illogical but may indeed be harmful.

Miscellaneous indications

In the past, tonsillectomy has been advised for enuresis, mental retarda-tion, focal sepsis, loss of appetite, catarrh, enlargement of cervical glands and asthma. There is no justification for the operation in these circum-stances.

Technique of tonsillectomy

The tonsils are usually removed by dissection under general endotra-cheal anaesthetic. Tonsillectomy used to be carried out by means of a guillotine under a short general anaesthetic, but this method does not allow the bleeding points to be tied and has now largely been given up. The adenoids are usually removed at the same time.

Nursing care

A child who has had its tonsils removed should be nursed for the first twelve hours on its side with its head down so that any blood will run out of the mouth and not down its trachea. Bleeding will also thus be obvious to the nursing staff.

The child should be observed for bleeding, and a half-hourly pulse chart should be kept for the first twelve hours. A rising pulse rate and/or bleeding should be reported immediately to the doctor.

General care

Pyrexia

Many patients have a slight fever the day after operation. This is a normal reaction to surgical trauma. It does not mean that the child should be given antibiotics and it can usually be expected to settle spontaneously.

Sore throat

These children obviously have a sore throat and may be unwilling to eat because of this. It is important, therefore, to encourage them to take an adequate diet, particularly of fluids. This symptom is often worse in the first few days after the patient has returned home.

Earache

Many patients complain of earache after tonsillectomy. This is usually a referred pain mediated by the glossopharyngeal nerve from the traumatised tonsillar fossa and is only rarely due to middle ear infection. Only simple analgesics are necessary for this pain.

Complications

The most important complication after tonsillectomy is haemorrhage, which may be primary, reactionary or secondary. Every year a few children die of post-tonsillectomy haemorrhage, usually reactionary, and often one of the factors leading to the patient's death is lack of awareness by junior medical and nursing staff of the potential seriousness of this complication. From a practical point of view, primary and reactionary haemorrhage can be considered together.

(a) *Primary and reactionary haemorrhage* appear in the first few hours after operation. It is the duty of the nursing staff to watch for this complication, and any bleeding, other than the most trivial, or a rise in pulse rate, should be reported without delay to the surgeon in charge of the operation.

Treatment

If bleeding is established, the child must be returned to theatre, the bleeding point found and tied. Other manoeuvres such as packing are usually useless and merely waste time and allow the child to lose more blood. Similarly, the old-fashioned practice of sedating the child with nepenthe is extremely dangerous, as the bleeding often continues unsuspected. Before returning the child to theatre, blood should be crossmatched, as by this time a child may have lost enough blood to be on the verge of shock. Also, the anaesthetic for this procedure must be given by a competent and experienced anaesthetist as these children often vomit large amounts of blood immediately after induction of anaesthetic. Once anaesthesia is induced, the bleeding point should be found and ligated.

(*b*) *Secondary haemorrhage* occurs about seven to ten days after operation. It is caused by infection.

Treatment

The amount of blood lost is almost always small and replacement is rarely required. Attempts to tie the bleeding point are unnecessary and indeed impossible as there is merely oozing from a granulating surface. The infection should be treated by penicillin.

Tonsillitis in adults

Attacks of tonsillitis usually end at puberty. Occasionally young adults also suffer this disease, but the systemic upset is usually less than in a child and a high fever seldom occurs. An attack of tonsillitis in an adult is more likely to be complicated by a quinsy than in a child.

Tonsillitis in an adult should be treated in the same way as in a child. It is important for an adult to stay in *bed* for several days; if he gets up too soon the attack is likely to recur.

Tonsillitis in a young adult should not be confused with a persistent sore throat due to chronic pharyngitis. In this disease there is no dysphagia or pyrexia. The common causes of chronic pharyngitis are bad teeth, smoking and mouth-breathing caused by nasal polypi, a deflected nasal septum or sepsis of the nose and sinuses.

Tonsillectomy seldom needs to be carried out in an adult and should only be done if there are frequently recurring attacks causing absence from work, or if the patient has had a quinsy. Tonsillitis over the age of forty-five is very uncommon, and such a diagnosis is almost certain to be wrong. A patient with throat symptoms over this age is much more likely to suffer from cancer.

ADENOIDS

The adenoid is a single pad of lymphoid tissue lying on the posterior wall of the nasopharynx. It is small at birth, begins to grow rapidly about the age of three, is maximal in size about the age of five and thereafter slowly atrophies, disappearing completely at puberty.

If this structure becomes very large it may block firstly the Eustachian tubes as they open into the nasopharynx, or secondly, the posterior apertures of the nose.

Obstruction of the Eustachian tube by an enlarged adenoid is a common cause of secretory otitis media (q.v.). Enlargement of the adenoid also causes stasis of secretions in the nasopharynx; infection can then readily occur and by extension up the Eustachian tubes cause acute otitis media.

Obstruction of the posterior apertures of the nose causes nasal obstruction. This results in mouth-breathing, and snoring at night. In addition, stasis of secretions in the nose may predispose to sinusitis.

If an enlarged adenoid is causing symptoms it should be removed. This is often done at the same time as tonsillectomy, the adenoids being removed by a curette.

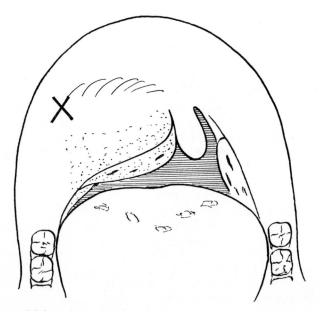

Fig. 41 Right quinsy, showing the uvula pushed across to the opposite side and point of incision to release pus.

QUINSY

Pathology

The tonsil is surrounded by a fascial space, the peri-tonsillar space. An attack of tonsillitis due to a particularly virulent strain of streptococci may spread beyond the tonsils, causing first cellulitis and later suppuration in this space.

Clinical features

Quinsy follows an acute attack of tonsillitis. About a week after the start of the original illness, the patient begins to feel unwell again and fever and dysphagia return. The characteristic symptom of quinsy is trismus; without this the diagnosis of quinsy is probably wrong. There is also referred pain to the ear on the same side. The diagram shows that the lateral relation of the peri-tonsillar space is the pterygoid muscles; trismus is caused by spread of oedema and infection from the space to these muscles.

The patient has difficulty in opening his mouth and the mouth is full of saliva because of dysphagia and trismus. The affected tonsil is displaced downwards and medially and there is a swelling above and lateral to the tonsil, the whole area being inflamed and oedematous. The uvula is also pushed to the opposite side and the palate is immobile.

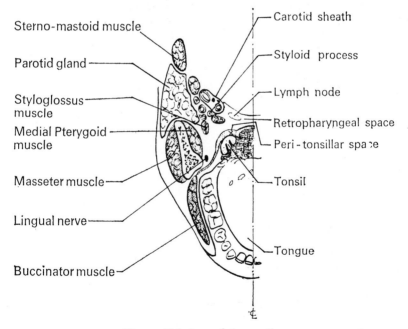

Fig. 42 Relations of the tonsil.

Treatment

In many patients when first seen, the disease has not progressed beyond the stage of cellulitis of the peri-tonsillar space. These patients can be expected to get better with large doses of intramuscular penicillin. If rapid resolution of symptoms and pyrexia does not occur within twenty-four hours the peri-tonsillar space should be drained. This is carried out under a local anaesthetic as a general anaesthetic in these circumstances is dangerous. Adequate anaesthesia can be produced by sucking a local anaesthetic lozenge of Amethocaine. The abscess is then drained by plunging a knife, whose point has been guarded by tape, into the anterior faucial pillar at the point shown in Figure 41. A swab should be obtained for culture and sensitivity and penicillin should be continued for a full seven days. The patient should also stay in bed until he feels fit to get up, usually about five to seven days.

A patient who has had a quinsy is likely to suffer from a recurrence, and because the peri-tonsillar space becomes obliterated by fibrous tissue the infection is likely to extend into the other fascial planes of the neck. Tonsillectomy should, therefore, be carried out six weeks after the attack.

Differential diagnosis
Retropharyngeal abscess and parapharyngeal abscess. Tumours of the tonsil particularly the reticuloses (q.v.). Mixed tumour ('pleomorphic adenoma') of the pharynx.

TUMOURS OF THE TONSIL

Benign tumours
Small papillomata often occur arising from the uvula or faucial pillars. They cause irritation of the throat and should be removed.

Other benign tumours are rare.

Malignant tumours
The tonsil consists of lymphoid tissue covered by squamous epithelium. Thus both reticuloses and squamous carcinoma occur at this site.

The reticuloses which occur here are lymphosarcoma and reticulum cell sarcoma. They occur at any age and present either with a unilateral swelling of the tonsil or with a gland in the neck. They are treated by radiotherapy.

Squamous carcinoma occurs most often about the age of sixty. It presents with a persistent sore throat, dysphagia and pain in the ear.

There is enlargement or ulceration of one tonsil and the corresponding jugulo-digastric node is usually enlarged.

This tumour is usually treated by radiotherapy; a recurrence is treated surgically as is an enlarged lymph node in the neck.

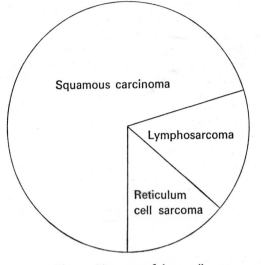

Fig. 43 Tumours of the tonsil.

Chapter Eighteen
Hoarseness

PHYSIOLOGY OF SPEECH

Speech is produced by two separate processes. A sound is produced by the larynx and is then modified by the lips, teeth, tongue and palate. The first process is called phonation, the second articulation.

During phonation the vocal cords must be able to meet along their entire length. If they do not, hoarseness, which is a roughness of the voice, is caused. It is to be distinguished from disorders of articulation and from aphonia, which is complete loss of the voice.

Hoarseness is the most important symptom of laryngeal disease. It always originates in the larynx, so that any patient who is hoarse must have something wrong with his larynx.

Normal apposition of the vocal cords during phonation may be prevented by oedema due to inflammation, by mechanical factors such as a tumour or by impaired mobility due to a lesion of the recurrent laryngeal nerve. A further cause of hoarseness is improper use of the voice, usually termed dysphonia. Some guidance as to the possible cause of hoarseness may be obtained from the history. If the patient suffers from inflammation of his larynx the disease will usually be short-lived and accompanied by the symptoms and signs of inflammation—fever, malaise, etc. If the patient has a tumour, however, there is no systemic upset and the hoarseness persists; indeed, it becomes worse with the passage of time.

Any doctor who does not have special training in examination of the ear, nose and throat should never forget that he cannot examine the larynx in such a way as to be able to give a patient a reliable opinion as to the cause of his hoarseness; furthermore, any patient over the age of forty who has hoarseness for more than two weeks must be presumed to have laryngeal cancer until conclusively proved otherwise.

INFLAMMATION

Acute laryngitis
Pathology
Any infection of the upper respiratory tract, due either to viruses or bacteria, often becomes generalised throughout the tract so that acute laryngitis often develops after a common cold. There is diffuse inflam-

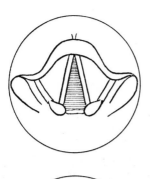

Quiet respiration

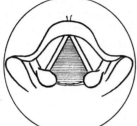

Deep inspiration

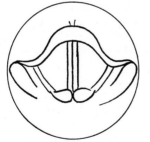

Phonation

Fig. 44 Positions of vocal cords compared.

mation of the entire laryngeal mucosa and oedema of its lax parts above and below the vocal cords. In a young child this mucosal swelling may cause respiratory obstruction. Pathogenic bacteria often cannot be isolated in these patients.

Clinical features
Acute laryngitis is an inflammatory disease. Its symptoms and signs are therefore those of inflammation. The most obvious symptom is hoarseness which may progress to aphonia. There is also fever,

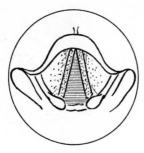

Inflammation

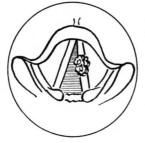

Tumour

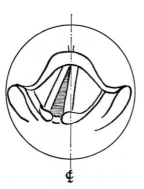

Paralysis
{The mobile cord can
sometimes cross over
the midline}

Fig. 45 Causes of hoarseness.

malaise, pain on speaking, and redness and swelling of the larynx. The disease is short-lived—four or five days. This differs completely from the otherwise symptomless hoarseness caused by an early tumour of the larynx.

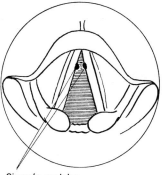

Singer's nodules

Fig. 46 Singer's nodules.

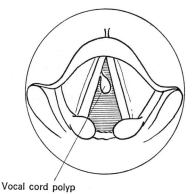

Vocal cord polyp

Fig. 47 Vocal cord polyp.

Investigations

The larynx should be examined with a mirror, when redness and swelling will be seen. The swelling affects particularly the parts above and below the vocal cords where the mucosa is not bound down.

Acute laryngitis is often associated with acute inflammation of the nose, sinuses or chest. The nose is therefore examined for pus and for inflammation of the mucosa. The chest and sinuses are X-rayed and a nasal and throat swab taken.

Treatment

1 Rest

An attack of acute laryngitis will resolve spontaneously if the larynx is put at rest. The patient must, therefore, use his voice little or not at all for two or three days; he should remain in a warm humid atmosphere and preferably in bed. He must not smoke or drink alcohol and must stay off work for a week to prevent too early resumption of use of his voice.

2 Antibiotics

Treatment with antibiotics is seldom indicated unless there is evidence of descending infection into the lower respiratory tract.

Chronic non-specific laryngitis

Aetiology

The larynx separates the upper from the lower respiratory tract. It may therefore be affected by disease from above or from below.

The commonest disorders of the upper respiratory tract associated with chronic laryngitis are chronic sinusitis, nasal polypi and a severely deflected nasal septum. In all these conditions there may be a discharge passing down the back of the nose to irritate the larynx; they also cause mouth-breathing which irritates the larynx.

The commonest disorder of the lower respiratory tract associated with chronic laryngitis is chronic bronchitis.

Pathology
Chronic inflammation of the larynx affects the entire laryngeal mucosa, which becomes diffusely inflamed, red and thickened. Histological examination in such cases very often shows areas of squamous metaplasia and these areas may become malignant.

Clinical features
Persistent hoarseness is usually the only symptom of chronic laryngitis. Dysphagia, pain in the throat and pain referred to the ear do not occur. A typical patient with chronic laryngitis is a middle-aged man with a red face and short neck who smokes and drinks heavily; often has chronic bronchitis, chronic sinusitis or carious teeth and has to shout at work. In taking a history from such a patient it is therefore important to enquire about his work and social habits, and about symptoms of nasal sepsis and of chest disease.

Investigations
Examination of the larynx shows the entire laryngeal mucosa to be red and thickened. The nose and nasopharynx are examined for sepsis, polypi or deflection of the nasal septum and the teeth for caries; an X-ray of the chest and sinuses must also be taken. If there is any doubt about the nature of the local disease of the larynx, an examination under anaesthetic and biopsy must be carried out.

Treatment
Diffuse chronic laryngitis is often secondary to disease of the nose or of the chest. Sinusitis should be treated, nasal polypi removed and a grossly deflected nasal septum resected if it is causing mouth breathing. Chronic bronchitis should be treated medically in an attempt to eradicate the purulent sputum which irritates the larynx. Removal of carious teeth often produces considerable improvement in these patients.

However, chronic diffuse laryngitis is often a penalty either of a patient's chest disease or a consequence of his way of life. Therefore, treatment is more likely to be rewarding if it is approached from the point of view of excluding malignancy as the cause of hoarseness rather than from the point of view of attempting to cure the chronic laryngitis.

Chronic specific laryngitis

Tuberculous

A. *Pathology*
Tuberculosis of the larynx is always secondary to pulmonary tuberculosis. Infected sputum causes ulceration of the larynx, affecting those parts which most come in contact with sputum, that is the inter-arytenoid space, the arytenoids and the ary-epiglottic folds. Usually the laryngeal lesion is on the same side as the infected lung.

B. *Clinical features*
In addition to being hoarse, the patient often has dysphagia, pain on swallowing and pain referred to the ear, because of ulceration of the pharynx. He is unwell, has lost weight and has a productive cough.

The patient may or may not be known to be suffering from pulmonary tuberculosis so that hoarseness may occasionally be the presenting symptom of pulmonary tuberculosis.

Indirect examination of the larynx with a mirror reveals the ulcerated areas of the inter-arytenoid space, arytenoids and the ary-epiglottic folds. There may be glands palpable in the neck. The local appearances may closely resemble those of carcinoma of the larynx.

C. *Treatment*
The pulmonary tuberculosis is treated with appropriate chemotherapy. The only specific therapy required for the larynx is voice rest. The progress should be followed by indirect laryngoscopy. With this treatment the lesion should heal in four weeks; if not, a coincident carcinoma should be suspected.

Syphilitic
Syphilitic laryngitis is now rarely seen in this country. The most common form is gummatous laryngitis, which is clinically indistinguishable from carcinoma. Therefore all patients before being treated for carcinoma of the larynx should have serological tests for syphilis.

Hyperkeratosis
Hyperkeratosis is a condition in which areas of keratinised squamous epithelium occur on the vocal cords.

The cause of this condition is unknown. The only symptom of it is hoarseness of long-standing. Examination of the larynx shows a white patch, usually on one vocal cord.

Hyperkeratosis is treated by removing the involved area endoscopically. These patients must be kept under observation by a laryngologist because malignant change sometimes occurs.

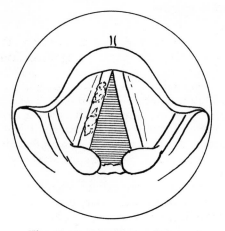

Fig. 48 Hyperkeratosis of larynx.

Dysphonia

This term is used to describe hoarseness resulting from misuse of the voice. There are many different types of dysphonia described, and indeed this forms the bulk of the study of the subject of phoniatrics. Dysphonias can however be divided for simplicity into hyperkinetic and hypokinetic. The latter is more often called hysterical aphonia in which there is complete loss of the voice, usually occurring in young women. There is no actual hoarseness, the voice either disappearing entirely or being replaced by a whisper. The patient can, however, cough.

Examination with a laryngeal mirror shows the vocal cords to spring apart on attempted phonation. No other abnormality of the larynx can be found. There is no organic cause for this lesion and it is a manifestation of hysteria. Complete recovery with speech therapy usually takes place; psychiatric advice may be necessary.

Hyperkinetic dysphonia occurs typically in the aggressive middle aged executive type, who uses his voice a lot at work, and is always under tension. Examination of the larynx in such a patient may show hypertrophy of the false cords (dysphonia plica ventricularis) or nodules on both vocal cords (singer's nodes). These nodules are often stated to occur at the junction of the anterior and middle thirds of the vocal cord; in fact they occur at the middle of the vibrating part of the vocal cord, which forms the anterior two thirds of the glottis. The middle of the vibrating cord is obviously the part most under strain.

This latter disorder is treated by a speech therapist, who gives instruction in correct breathing and speech production techniques. The nodules may need to be removed endoscopically.

TUMOURS

Benign

True benign tumours of the larynx are uncommon. Papillomata occur in children and are multiple, whereas a single papillomata is occasionally seen in adults. These tumours cause hoarseness and stridor in children (q.v.); they should be removed via an endoscope with forceps. Chondromas and haemangiomas occur rarely. They cause hoarseness, and because of their size may cause stridor. They should be removed, if small, endoscopically; if large, by an external incision.

Nodules of the vocal cords are not true tumours but are usually collections of oedematous tissue caused by hyperkinetic dysphonia (q.v.).

Polyps

A vocal cord polyp occurs typically on one vocal cord arising from the middle of the vibrating part of one vocal cord. Its cause is uncertain but it may be due to misuse of the voice.

The polyp is removed endoscopically, and if necessary the patient is sent to a speech therapist to correct vocal abuse.

Malignant

A. Carcinoma of the larynx
Pathology

For the purposes of description of tumours the larynx is divided into three anatomical areas, the supraglottis, the glottis and the subglottis. Tumours of the supraglottic and subglottic areas must be quite large before they involve the vocal cords and produce hoarseness. They thus tend to present fairly late. Also they occur in areas of rich lymphatic drainage and many patients with these tumours have a palpable lymph gland in the neck when first seen. Tumours of the true vocal cords, however, present early, usually when the cord is still mobile. The vocal cords have a poor lymphatic drainage and these patients do not develop metastases to lymph nodes.

Virtually all malignant tumours of the larynx are squamous cell carcinomas.

Symptoms

Hoarseness is the presenting symptom of carcinoma of the larynx. It is also the ONLY symptom of this disease for many months. Unlike the hoarseness of laryngitis, it is not accompanied by systemic symptoms such as fever, it persists and becomes worse over several weeks or months. There are no other symptoms until the disease is far advanced, by which time stridor occurs because of respiratory obstruction. If the tumour extends beyond the larynx to invade the pharynx, the patient complains of dysphagia, pain on swallowing and pain referred to the ear.

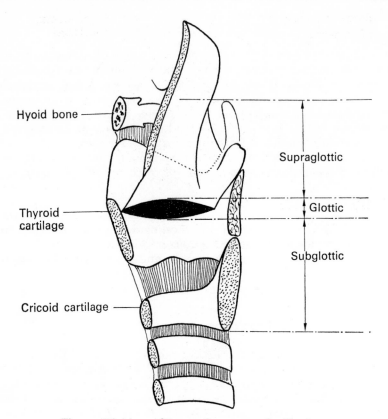

Fig. 49 Divisions of Larynx for tumour classification.

Signs
Until the late stage of the disease there are no signs of carcinoma of the larynx which can be elicited by a doctor who cannot use a laryngeal mirror. In the later stage an enlarged lymph gland may be felt in the neck, and occasionally the tumour may be felt, causing expansion of the larynx. If the patient is to be given a reasonable chance of successful treatment, however, the disease must be diagnosed before this stage. Therefore, any patient who is hoarse for more than two weeks must be referred to a competent laryngologist without delay.

Investigations
In addition to the history of his hoarseness the patient should be asked about his general health, his occupation and whether he smokes, as these factors influence his treatment.
Examination of the larynx with a laryngeal mirror will reveal the tumour; the common sites are shown in the diagram. The patient's

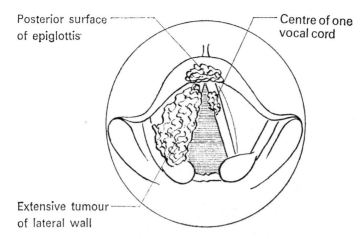

Posterior surface of epiglottis

Centre of one vocal cord

Extensive tumour of lateral wall

Fig. 50 Common sites of laryngeal tumours.

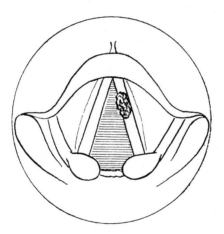

Fig. 51 Tumour confined to one vocal cord.

general health should be assessed by an X-ray of the chest, sputum culture, E.C.G. and haemoglobin estimation. The larynx is then examined under anaesthesia and a portion of the tumour taken for biopsy. Carious teeth are removed at the same time.

Treatment

Unless there is a distant metastasis, which is rare, almost all patients with laryngeal cancer are suitable for treatment with the exception that a very old patient is sometimes better left alone.

The two possible forms of treatment are surgery and radiotherapy. Radiotherapy has the advantage of preserving a normal voice but

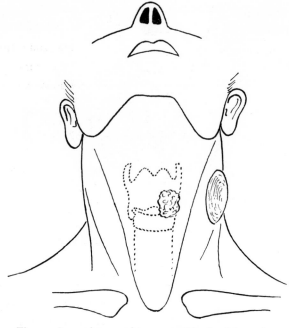

Fig. 52 Large laryngeal tumour with gland in neck.

seldom cures an advanced tumour, particularly if associated with enlarged lymph nodes. Radiotherapy should, therefore, be used for the patient with a small lesion with no enlarged lymph nodes. The ideal case is a tumour confined to one vocal cord which is still mobile. Nine out of ten of such patients will be permanently cured by radiotherapy and will retain their voice. Fixation of the vocal cord indicates spread of the disease to invade the muscle layers. If the tumour has not spread to the supra- or sub-glottic area, this lesion can still be treated with radiotherapy but with a poorer prognosis. If the tumour recurs, total laryngectomy should be carried out.

A patient with a large laryngeal tumour, associated with enlarged lymph nodes, is best treated by total laryngectomy and block dissection of the glands of the neck. This applies to tumours of the sub- and supra-glottic groups. In these patients the chance of cure is not so high; one patient in three will be cured permanently.

B. *After-care of the laryngectomee*

After a laryngectomy most patients need extensive rehabilitation. They must be taught oesophageal speech by a speech therapist. They need retraining because heavy work is difficult after this operation, but many patients return to heavy labouring jobs.

As these patients have a permanent tracheostomy, they usually need

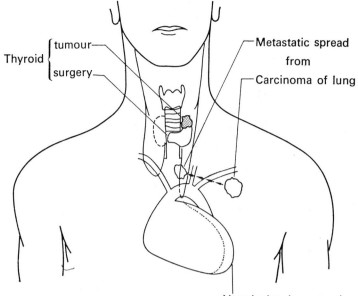

Thyroid { tumour—
{ surgery—

Metastatic spread
from
Carcinoma of lung

Ventricular hypertrophy, with
unfolding of aortic arch,
causing traction on the left
recurrent laryngeal nerve

Fig. 53 Causes of hoarseness from nerve paralysis.

to wear a tracheostomy tube, although many can do without one after a few months, perhaps sleeping with a tube in place to prevent contraction of the stoma.

As inspired air is no longer breathed through the nose, crusting of the trachea due to inhalation of dry air is sometimes a problem. This can be overcome by sleeping with a humidifier in the bedroom.

Perhaps most important of all is that these patients need reassurance and encouragement to lead a normal life.

NEUROLOGICAL DISEASES

Recurrent laryngeal nerve palsy

Besides inflammation and tumour formation, hoarseness may also be caused by interference with the normal movements of the vocal cords.

The vocal cords are moved by several muscles within the cartilaginous framework of the larynx. They can be arranged into two groups: those which abduct the vocal cords away from the midline and those which adduct the vocal cords towards the midline. There is no point in the undergraduate attempting to remember the names of the individual

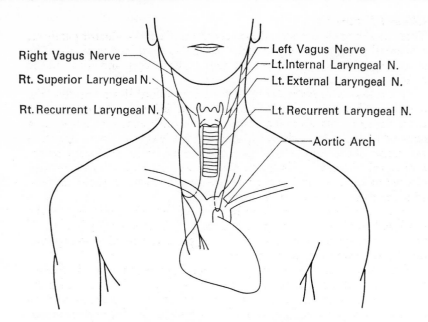

Right Vagus Nerve

Rt. Superior Laryngeal N.

Rt. Recurrent Laryngeal N.

Left Vagus Nerve
Lt. Internal Laryngeal N.
Lt. External Laryngeal N.
Lt. Recurrent Laryngeal N.
Aortic Arch

Fig. 54 Course of right and left vagus nerves.

muscles. Both these muscle groups are supplied by the recurrent laryngeal nerve which arises from the vagus nerve so that a laryngeal paralysis may be caused by a lesion of either nerve.

A lesion of the vagus or recurrent laryngeal nerves may be incomplete or may be complete from the start.

In an incomplete lesion of the vagus or recurrent laryngeal nerves only the abductor group of muscles are paralysed so that the vocal cord becomes fixed in or near the midline. If such a lesion progresses, or if the lesion is complete from the start, all the muscles become paralysed and the vocal cord becomes fixed in a half-way position known as the cadaveric position. This curious phenomenon has never been satisfactorily explained since it was first described by Semon.

Tension of the vocal cord is also controlled by a muscle on the outside of the laryngeal framework, the crico-thyroid muscle, which is supplied by the external laryngeal nerve. Isolated lesions of this nerve are rare and will not be considered further.

The right and left recurrent laryngeal nerves run different courses, the right arising in the root of the neck and the left arising in the mediastinum at the arch of the aorta. A paralysis on the right side is therefore caused by a lesion of the vagus or recurrent laryngeal nerve in the neck. On the left side either nerve may be affected either in the neck or in the superior mediastinum.

Clinical features

Three common clinical situations occur: a unilateral abductor paralysis, a bilateral abductor paralysis and a unilateral complete paralysis. The causes, symptoms, signs and treatment of each vary and they will be considered separately.

In a *unilateral abductor paralysis* the affected cord lies at or near the midline. This lesion usually occurs on the left side, the commonest cause being pressure on the vagus or recurrent laryngeal nerve by a mass of malignant glands in the superior mediastinum, secondary to a carcinoma of the lung. Hoarseness may indeed be the presenting symptom in this disease. This lesion may also be seen occasionally in carcinoma of the thyroid gland or oesophagus and after thyroid surgery. In some patients the cause is never found.

The other vocal cord is fully mobile and approximates to the paralysed cord on phonation. Thus the patient may not be hoarse. If he is hoarse, spontaneous recovery takes place as a result of compensation by the other mobile vocal cord.

Examination in this lesion shows one vocal cord to be immobile and lying in the midline; the arytenoid cartilage falls forward on the same side. The larynx must always be examined under anaesthesia to exclude other causes of fixation of the vocal cord. The arytenoid and the cord are also tested for mobility to distinguish a vocal cord palsy from an arthrodesis of the crico-arytenoid joint. In a palsy the arytenoid and cord can be moved by the laryngoscope. In arthrodesis of the joint, usually due to rheumatoid arthritis, the arytenoid is fixed.

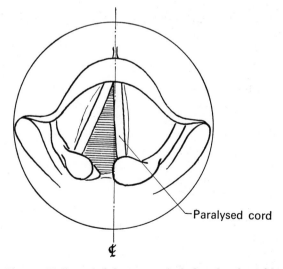

Paralysed cord

Fig. 55 Unilateral abductor paralysis (paralysed cord in, or close to, the centre line).

No treatment is required for this condition as spontaneous compensation usually takes place. In the majority of patients this lesion is caused by a carcinoma of the lung; paralysis of one vocal cord is a contra-indication to surgery in this condition so that the patient has not long to live in any case.

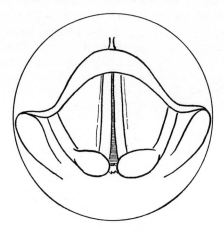

Fig. 56 Bilateral abductor paralysis.

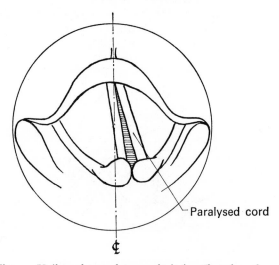

Fig. 57 Unilateral complete paralysis (unaffected cord can often cross over the centre line).

A *bilateral abductor paralysis* is uncommon. It is usually seen after operations on the thyroid gland. Both vocal cords are paralysed in or near the midline. Because of this the voice may be quite good but the most obvious symptom is stridor, so that a tracheostomy is necessary. Such a patient may need to wear a tracheostomy permanently. A satisfactory airway can be produced, however, by an operation called a chordopexy in which one vocal vord is fixed away from the midline. The voice may be rough after this operation and it should not be advised for a patient who depends on his voice for his living.

A *unilateral complete paralysis* indicates complete paralysis of the recurrent laryngeal nerve. This is usually caused by surgery either of the thyroid gland or during thoracotomy. The vocal cord becomes paralysed away from the midline, leaving a gap between the cords. The other cord is usually unable to compensate for this and the patient becomes extremely hoarse due to air waste during attempted phonation. Even worse, he may inhale his food and suffer repeated chest infections. This lesion can be treated very simply by injecting Teflon into the paralysed cord to increase its bulk so that the opposite cord strikes against it during phonation.

Chapter Nineteen
Dysphagia

INTRODUCTION
Swallowing occurs in three stages. The first stage occurs in the mouth, where a bolus of food is prepared by the teeth and tongue and propelled backwards into the pharynx. In the second stage, the orifices leading from the pharynx close, except for the oesophageal opening which relaxes; the bolus is propelled through it into the oesophagus. During the third stage a peristaltic wave carries the bolus down the oesophagus; when it reaches the bottom of the oesophagus the cardia relaxes and the food enters the stomach.

While strictly speaking the term dysphagia should only be used to describe interference by an organic lesion to the passage of the bolus through the oesophagus, there are many other diseases in which the patient's first complaint is of difficulty in swallowing, therefore all these diseases will be discussed here, and an attempt made to show how some of these can be recognised from the patient's history.

Despite the long list of causes of dysphagia given in this and other books, the doctor must always have foremost in his mind that a patient who has had difficulty in swallowing *solid* food for two weeks or more has cancer of the pharynx or oesophagus until proved otherwise.

PHARYNGEAL DISEASE

Acute tonsillitis and pharyngitis
Acute inflammation in the mouth or pharynx is accompanied by difficulty in deglutition. The commonest disease is, of course, acute tonsillitis in which there is also a fever and malaise, but the disease lasts a few days only.

Chronic pharyngitis
Chronic pharyngitis is always secondary to disease of surrounding organs and is a common cause of persistent sore throat; it does not, however, cause difficulty in swallowing food, though it may cause a feeling of a persistent lump in the throat.

The common causes of pharyngeal irritation are excessive smoking, dental sepsis, and mouth-breathing due to sinusitis, a deflected nasal septum or nasal polypi. These should be treated appropriately.

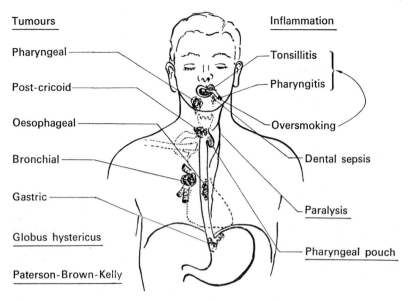

Fig. 58 Causes of dysphagia.

'A lump in the throat'

A feeling of a lump in the throat is a common complaint. The patient is usually a middle-aged woman who complains of a persistent feeling of a lump in the throat, which is more noticeable when she swallows saliva but does not interfere in any way with the swallowing of food. There are no other symptoms, no hoarseness, no sore throat and no loss of weight.

This condition is often called 'globus hystericus' and while it is true that the condition may be due to spasm of the upper oesophageal sphincter, many of these patients have reflux oesophagitis.

This diagnosis should *never be made* if the patient has difficulty in swallowing solid food; such a patient has cancer until proved otherwise.

Carcinoma of the pharynx

Virtually all tumours of the pharynx are squamous cell carcinomas. Unlike other carcinomas of the head and neck, carcinomas of the pharynx are commoner in women and occur at a younger age and may even be seen in women as young as twenty-five. Some patients with these tumours have a history of the Paterson-Brown-Kelly syndrome (p. 129).

These tumours often extend into the larynx; the patient then becomes hoarse. She may also have earache because the ear and the

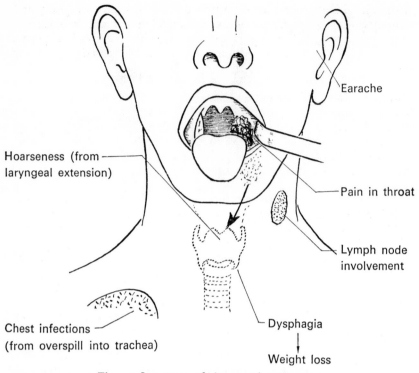

Earache

Hoarseness (from
laryngeal extension)

Pain in throat

Lymph node
involvement

Chest infections
(from overspill into trachea)

Dysphagia

Weight loss

Fig. 59 Symptoms of pharyngeal carcinoma.

pharynx have a common sensory nerve supply from the glosso pharyn-geal and the vagus nerves.

Loss of weight inevitably occurs in these patients as their difficulty in swallowing food increases. Often a patient will have lost twenty to thirty pounds (9 to 14 kg) in weight; this amount of weight loss in-volves loss of protein as well as fat. Loss of body protein to this extent has a profound effect on healing, and attention to this is a vital factor in the treatment of these patients.

In the later stages, spill-over into the trachea occurs so that the patient suffers recurrent, or chronic, chest infections. In addition to examination of the larynx and pharynx with a mirror and palpation of the neck, any patient with difficulty in swallowing food localised to the pharynx should have a barium swallow and an oesophagoscopy.

Occasionally, the barium swallow may be reported as normal, but if the patient's symptoms are real a negative report should be ignored and an oesophagoscopy carried out. The tumour can be seen, its extent assessed and a specimen taken for biopsy.

The possible forms of treatment of these tumours are surgery or radiotherapy. Because these tumours are large and are often associated with enlarged lymph nodes the results of radiotherapy are poor, and surgery gives a better chance of saving the patient's life. The operation requires removal of both the larynx and the pharynx; the latter must be reconstituted either by skin flaps or by the transposed stomach or colon.

Paterson–Brown-Kelly syndrome

This disease was first described in Britain by Paterson and Brown-Kelly and was described a short time later in the United States by Plummer and Vinson. It occurs in middle-aged women and is characterised by glossitis, anaemia, dysphagia and koilonychia. It is an uncommon disease of unknown cause but is important because it is precancerous.

The mucosa of the pharynx, mouth and oesophagus become atrophied and glazed, and there are often fissures at the angle of the mouth. A fibrous stricture forms, usually at the upper end of the oesophagus. This appears typically as a web on a barium swallow.

The patient is obviously anaemic and shows the stigmata of long-standing microcytic anaemia, such as koilonychia.

An oesophagoscopy should always be carried out. This allows a stricture to be dilated, and malignant change detected.

Investigation of the blood shows a microcytic anaemia with a low serum iron. There is also achlorhydria of the stomach.

Treatment

The anaemia should be treated by oral iron and the dysphagia, due to web formation, should be relieved by dilatation. The patient must be kept under observation because malignant change may occur. The commonest site for a carcinoma to occur is the post-cricoid area, but this disease may precede any tumour of the pharynx or oesophagus.

Pharyngeal paralysis

The muscles of the pharynx are supplied by the vagus nerve and the cranial root of the accessory nerve. Lesions of these nerves, particularly if bilateral, cause dysphagia. The common causes include pseudobulbar palsy, bulbar poliomyelitis, upper motor neurone disease, and carcinoma of the nasopharynx invading the base of the skull. Myasthenia gravis can also cause, or even present with, dysphagia.

Usually these lesions are fundamentally untreatable, and often the best that can be hoped for is to feed the patient adequately, and protect his trachea from over-spill of food and saliva. A gastrostomy and a tracheostomy may thus be needed.

Foreign bodies in the pharynx and oesophagus

Patients at any age may suffer an impaction of a foreign body in the pharynx or oesophagus. Children often swallow coins and other round objects while playing; young adults, because they usually have their own teeth, do not swallow large hard objects but may get fish bones stuck in their tonsils; older patients, because they do not have their own teeth, often do not chew their food properly and swallow meat bones.

The presence of the foreign body irritates the gullet so that the patient makes repeated and futile attempts at swallowing and in an attempt to wash the foreign body downwards excess saliva is produced. Because of the irritation produced by the foreign body the patient usually localises it well.

Impacted foreign bodies are dangerous because they produce laceration of the delicate mucosa leading to a para-pharyngeal or peri-oesophageal abscess. These are dangerous, particularly the latter which causes death from mediastinitis.

A patient who says that he has swallowed a foreign body, particularly if he can localise it and is producing a lot of frothy saliva, should be treated by an emergency oesophagoscopy to remove the foreign body. This must be done carefully, particularly in the case of meat bones as they can easily tear the mucosa.

OESOPHAGEAL DISEASE

Introduction
Dysphagia due to interference with the transmission of the food along the oesophagus, should be distinguished from the difficulties of deglutition produced by bulbar lesions, myasthenia gravis and hypochromic anaemias where there is a weakness of propulsion of food through the pharynx, so that there is difficulty in actually getting the bolus to the oesophagus.

In oesophageal dysphagia the patient complains that the food is held up at some level in the thorax, which he can frequently locate quite accurately. In most cases it is solid food which first gives rise to difficulty, and this may proceed to total obstruction even for fluids. Substernal discomfort is noted first as the food is held up and oesophageal peristalsis increases to force it through the narrowed area. These contractions become more severe, giving rise to substernal pain which may be acute, radiating to the back and up into the neck and angles of the jaws on both sides. Relief is obtained by regurgitation or by passage of the bolus through the obstruction. In some cases of cardiospasm, patients find that there is more difficulty with fluids than with solids, probably due to the solid material causing more stimulation to relax the lower oesophagus than do fluids.

Total obstruction of the oesophagus produces an intolerable state whereby the lumen fills with fluid or saliva, which then spills over into the larynx and down the trachea, producing continuous coughing, hawking and spluttering, causing great distress to the patient.

Some dilatation of the oesophagus occurs above the obstruction in course of time, with considerable muscular hypertrophy, but it is never as great as the enormous distension that can occur with cardiospasm where the oesophageal lumen can reach a diameter of ten centimetres or more, associated with the progressive muscular paralysis of the organ.

Tracheo-oesophageal fistula

Dysphagia may present in the first few hours of life in association with a congenital tracheo-oesophageal fistula. The baby, after sucking or taking fluids, splutters, coughs and regurgitates the material taken in, due to overfilling of the blind upper oesophageal pouch causing spill-over into the lungs. After forty-eight hours progressive broncho-pneumonia develops and it is essential to recognise the condition before this time. The passage of a soft catheter through the mouth is inter-rupted after some inches and the injection of one millilitre of radio-opaque oil will demonstrate the presence of the upper oesophageal pouch. Immediate anastomosis of the two ends of the oesophagus with closure of the tracheal fistula is performed, curing two-thirds of these patients. Occasional dilatation of the site of oesophageal anasta-mosis may be required if there is a residual stricture.

Caustic burns of the oesophagus

This accident is included because immediate treatment by a casualty officer can give great relief and minimise the later development of an oesophageal stricture.

Children sometimes swallow caustic fluids; they are brought into hospital, severely shocked, complaining of pain in the chest and in-ability to swallow saliva. Examination of the lips and mouth demon-strates the severity of the chemical burn which is taking place in the oesophagus. The areas most severely involved are the region of the upper oesophageal sphincter, the arch of the aorta and the cardiac sphincter, for here the fluid tends to be transiently held up, due to spasm of the oesophageal muscle. Exfoliation of the mucosa takes place with severe oedema and ulceration of the oesophageal wall, and may be of the stomach also. As the specific chemical neutraliser is usually unavailable, and in the emotional disturbance the story from the relatives is often unreliable, the passage of a stomach tube and a good wash-out with tap water is the most convenient emergency treat-ment. Shock is then treated and swallowing must be forbidden for at least ten days. The fluid and nutritional balance can be maintained in-travenously for a time but a gastrostomy is frequently necessary after a week. Steroid therapy should be started from the beginning to minimise fibrous tissue formation during the healing process. After seven to ten days, oesophagoscopy is performed to study the state of the oesophagus and allow bouginage of any strictured area. This can be repeated frequently after this time, eventually establishing a 'rail-road' of a string passing through the oesophagus, out through the gastrostomy opening, and back into the mouth. A bougie tied to this string is a useful method of performing a frequent dilatation of the stricture, which the child may learn to do himself. Perseverance with bouginage over a long period of time can be very rewarding as many of the strictures soften in time. If, however, long areas of narrowing persist, then an oesophagectomy with colon replacement may be required in the end.

Spasm of the oesophagus
By virtue of a very extensive nerve plexus which surrounds and ramifies through it, the oesophagus is easily induced to go into spasm. The onset of multiple areas of spasm, often associated with quite severe substernal pain and dysphagia, tends to occur with emotional factors—the

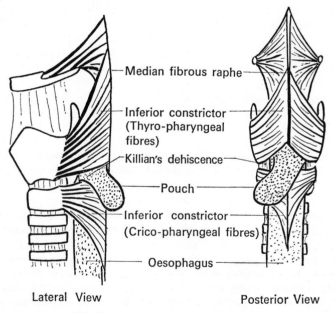

Lateral View   Posterior View

Fig. 60 Genesis of pharyngeal pouch.

'Corkscrew oesophagus'. The tortuous contraction of the oesophagus produces a characteristic appearance on barium swallow. No treatment is available other than reassurance that the disease is benign. Spasm of the upper and lower sphincter areas is responsible for the development of diverticula above them. The pharyngeal diverticulum occurs through a weak portion in the midline, posteriorly, of the inferior constrictor muscle and consists essentially of a herniation of the mucosa with a few stretched muscle fibres over it. It becomes dependent and the patient complains of difficulty in passing food into the oesophagus together with a swelling developing in the lower part of the neck, usually on the left side and the regurgitation of undigested food into the mouth some hours after eating. Relief is obtained by excision of the pouch and a myotomy of the superior sphincter of the oesophagus. Similarly, a diverticulum can develop in the lower oesophagus above a spastic area—the epiphrenic diverticulum, which fills with food and presses on the oesophagus from without, giving a mild form of dysphagia. Treatment again is by excision of the diverticulum and a myotomy of the lower oesophagus. Traction diverticula of the oesophagus, resulting from attachment of the oesophageal wall to caseous tuberculous mediastinal glands, are usually inverted so that food does not collect in them and they do not cause dysphagia.

Achalasia

Cardiospasm or achalasia of the cardia is a spastic state of the lower end of the oesophagus which usually involves not only the cardiac 'sphincter' but also several centimetres of the lower oesophagus. Dysphagia in this condition almost invariably follows an acute emotional crisis. In the first place retention of food is intermittent, the oesophagus fills with food which may suddenly empty into the stomach or which may have to be vomited back to get relief of the substernal discomfort. Curiously the dysphagia may sometimes be more persistent with a fluid diet than with solids, as the stimulation of the solid material may cause relaxation of the lower oesophageal spasm. Once established, however, the condition seems to be permanent, and the rate of eating becomes progressively slower to permit relaxation of the oesophagus in between the delayed openings of the lower end. Progressive dilatation of the oesophagus occurs with loss of contractability and finally the organ becomes an inert sac in which stasis of food over long periods occurs, leading to ulceration and malignant change. Of all the procedures advocated for relief of this condition such as bouginage, hydrostatic dilators, oesophagogastrostomy and inhalation of octyl nitrite, none have given the permanent relief that can be obtained by undertaking a cardio-oesophago-myotomy (Heller's operation). Provided that the incision of the circular fibres of the contracted area of the oesophagus is carried well on to the dilated oesophagus above and the stomach below, full and permanent relief can be obtained in almost all patients.

Carcinoma of the oesophagus

The most common form of dysphagia, however, is that due to malignant disease of the oesophagus or cardiac end of the stomach. Patients usually seek advice about three months after they have noticed a transient difficulty in swallowing and at this stage are only able to take semi-solids and fluids. Blockage of the progressively narrowing stricture with solid food gives rise to severe substernal discomfort and pain in the back, and vomiting will be required to clear the oesophagus. Such patients usually have no previous history of swallowing difficulties or dysphagia. The size of the tumour depends upon its pathological nature, a small scirrhous type of neoplasm producing severe obstruction, while a papilliferous type of tumour may grow to a large size without severe symptoms; carcinoma of the oesophagus is on the whole a rapidly extending tumour and involvement of the neighbouring glands and particularly the coeliac axis group in middle and lower third tumours occurs early. Submucosal infiltration along the lymphatics also occurs early and this cannot be felt on palpation, so that if surgical excision is carried out the oesophagus must be divided at least eight centimetres above all palpable tumour.

Diagnosis is made by oesophagoscopy, and in the care of tumours of the middle and upper third of the oesophagus, bronchoscopy should also be performed to exclude involvement of the left bronchus or trachea.

Many of these patients are being progressively starved, and prior to operation it is important to be satisfied that the water balance, blood protein levels, haemoglobin and vitamin levels are within usual limits.

Surgical treatment is the method of choice for carcinoma of the middle and lower third of the oesophagus (squamous carcinoma) and the cardiac end of stomach (adenocarcinoma). The tumour, together with eight centimetres of the oesophagus above, a portion of the stomach below and the lymphatic field is removed *en bloc*, and in the case of carcinoma of the cardia, the spleen and greater omentum may also have to be excised in continuity. Alimentary continuity is re-established by anastomosing the lower end of the oesophagus to the upper end of the stomach. Some surgeons prefer to perform an oesophago-jejunal anastomosis or insert a colonic implant between the oesophagus and the stomach.

Surgery for carcinoma of the upper third of the oesophagus is not very satisfactory owing to the difficulties of excising adequately the lymphatic field which extends up into both sides of the neck; radiotherapy probably gives better palliation.

Many carcinomas of the oesophagus are potentially incurable by surgery when seen owing to involvement of the aorta, bronchial tree, liver metastases, etc. If the growth can be excised, this provides the best form of palliation, but occasionally an anastomosis can be made above the growth to the stomach or jejunum. The symptoms of progressive dysphagia leading to the stage of salivary regurgitation are so distressing that palliation by the insertion of a tube wherever possible should be undertaken. This may be possible via an oesophagoscope where a plastic or Souttar's tube is passed over a bougie inserted through the tumour, or by drawing a Mousseau-Barbin tube down through the growth from a small gastrostomy.

Benign oesophageal tumours

The common simple tumour of the oesophagus—the leiomyoma—can grow to a very large size as it arises from one side of the oesophagus and the oesophageal lumen enlarges around it. Dysphagia is consequently mild in this condition unless the end of the tumour impacts in the cardiac orifice.

Oesophageal strictures

Inflammatory strictures due to tuberculosis and syphilis have now virtually disappeared but they still occur in the Paterson–Brown-Kelly syndrome (q.v.).

Peptic stricture of the oesophagus secondary to reflex oesophagitis associated with a hiatus hernia can produce severe dysphagia but there is nearly always a long history of substernal discomfort, indigestion and heartburn prior to the difficulty in swallowing. With the onset of dysphagia the symptoms of oesophagitis often disappear as the regurgitation is minimised by the stricture. A high proportion of cases of peptic stricture occur in later life as more time is spent in bed, and probably the mucosal anti-acid defences become less potent. Repeated dilatation is helpful, but surgical treatment may be necessary. This includes an open dilatation of the stricture via the herniated end of the stomach and narrowing the oesophageal hiatus, or even an excision of the stricture with partial gastrectomy and myotomy. The development of a peptic stricture of the oesophagus is an indication that the surgical reduction of the hiatus hernia has been left too late, and what would have been a simple curative procedure has now become a formidable problem.

Miscellaneous causes of dysphagia

The oesophagus may be compressed from without, particularly by malignant glands from a bronchial carcinoma and dysphagia results requiring intubation. A mild degree of dysphagia may result from thyroid enlargement, cardiac enlargement, aneurysms and mediastinal tumours, but this is usually not severe and seldom requires special treatment of itself, and is usually cured if the cause of pressure can be removed.

'Dysphagia Lusoria' is due to an aberrant subclavian artery arising from the aortic arch distal to the left subclavian artery and passing across the mediastinum behind the oesophagus to the right arm. Symptoms usually arise in childhood and the patient has a 'hesitant' type of dysphagia. Barium swallow shows a narrowing of the posterior surface of the upper oesophagus and on oesophagoscopy pressure on the swelling, which is seen, causes obliteration of the right radial pulse. Division of the aberrant artery cures the condition.

Finally, when no clear organic causes of dysphagia can be found, examination for the presence of bulbar lesions causing deglutition disturbances should be undertaken.

Scleroderma of the oesophagus can cause difficulty in bolus transmission and this condition can be suspected when cutaneous manifestations are present.

It is axiomatic, however, to consider that 'dysphagia' as a symptom in an adult is due to a carcinoma until this has been eliminated. Preliminary investigation by a Barium swallow is simple and nearly always diagnostic, and should be performed without any delay.

Chapter Twenty
Stridor in childhood

DEFINITION
Stridor is a noise which indicates that there is obstruction to the passage of air, into or out of the lower respiratory tract; it is always an important symptom when it is heard in the adult or the child because obstructed breathing may call for the making of an artificial airway (tracheostomy), or for the introduction of an endotracheal tube. Many adults with stridor have other symptoms such as hoarseness, dyspnoea and cough, which warn the physician that there is a potentially serious situation in the lower respiratory tract. The baby and young child may have no other symptom and for this reason alone it is imperative that all children presenting with stridor should be examined, a diagnosis made, and the parents advised as to the course and the management of the condition. Stridor may be of three different kinds:

1 Inspiratory
This is a crowing noise colloquially called 'croup'. It has a quasi-musical quality. The cause is usually to be found in the larynx.

2 Expiratory
This is due to bronchial obstruction, and is usually called wheezing.

3 Two-way
This is a combination of the two preceding varieties, and the noises made are similar to, but not identical with, the two preceding noises. The obstruction usually lies in the trachea.

ANATOMY OF A BABY'S LARYNX
There are certain well-recognised differences between a baby's larynx and that of the adult.

1 The baby's larynx is both relatively and absolutely smaller than the adult's.
2 The baby's larynx lies higher in the neck and descends to the adult position during the first months of life.
3 The tissues of the baby's larynx are softer than those of the adult.
4 There is considerable variation in the ratio of the size of the glottis to the size of the child.

5 The mucosa covering the baby's larynx is hypersensitive; this is a protective mechanism to ensure that the baby's airway is protected against ill co-ordinated attempts at swallowing.

It is these differences which make the accurate diagnosis of the cause of the stridor so important.

CAUSES

The various lesions which cause stridor may be classified thus:

	Congenital			Acquired
	Functional	*Structural*		
Larynx	Paresis or Paralysis	Supra-glottic	Congenital laryngeal stridor	F.B. Inflammation
			Cysts Tumours	
		Glottic	Webs Tumours	
		Sub-glottic	Tumours or congenital Sub-glottic stenosis	
Trachea	Vascular ring	Congenital tracheal stenosis Absent tracheal rings		F.B. Inflammation
Bronchus	Asthma			F.B. Inflammation

CLINICAL APPROACH TO THE STRIDULOUS CHILD

The approach to any patient, we are taught, rests on a careful history followed by an equally careful clinical examination. This is perfectly true, but in the case of the stridulous child the history may have to be obtained from anxious or inexperienced parents, and may not in fact be of much real value in arriving at a diagnosis. There is however, one all-important question which every parent can answer, and this is 'How long has the noise been present'? From this it may be possible to gather what the child was doing at the time that the noise began—for example, he might have been eating peanuts! When acute inflammation is the cause of the obstruction, we are frequently told that the child went to bed at the normal time—perfectly well—only to wake up two hours later with noisy and disturbed breathing. If the stridor has been present since birth and the parents have become in some measure reconciled to the noise of it, it is of value to ask about cough, feeding difficulties and recurrent chest infections. Then too, enquiries should be made for failure to gain weight or loss of weight. The length and perfection of the history obtained must, however, be governed by the urgency of the situation; but however urgent the situation appears to

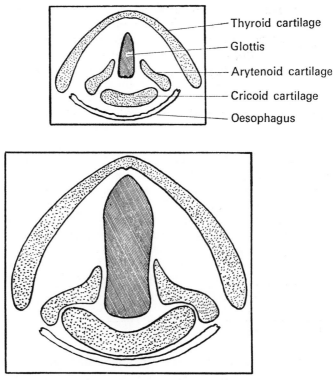

Infant

Thyroid cartilage

Glottis

Arytenoid cartilage

Cricoid cartilage

Oesophagus

Adult

Fig. 61 Cross section through glottis (approximately to scale). The glottis in infants is both relatively and absolutely smaller than in the adult (A–P diameters of glottis: infant 7 mm, Adult ♂ = 23 mm).

be, it is essential before any endoscopic examination is carried out that the child should be examined clinically; this examination can provide vital information as to the site of the obstruction.

Order of examination

1 Listen for the noise, and try to decide where it comes in respiratory cycle.
2 Has it a musical croupy quality?—Larynx. Has it a gruff tone with an added sound in expiration?—Tracheal. Has it a wheezy quality on expiration?—Bronchial.
3 Put your head to the baby's chest and try to clarify your first impression.
4 Turn the child into the prone position and see if the noise disappears, if it does not, then turn the child first to one side and then to the other. Does the noise disappear? If the noise does disappear, this suggests that the cause of the stridor lies in the

surrounding structures, rather than in the lumen of the larynx or trachea.

As it is essential that the diagnosis should be made at this point, a direct examination of the larynx and tracheo-bronchial tree must be made by the laryngologist; this can be carried out with complete safety if the anaesthetic is administered by a skilled children's anaesthetist. He will pass an endotracheal tube if he can and will keep the child oxygenated while a diagnosis is being made. The laryngologist in making a direct examination, is seeking information about the following points:

1 The size, shape and function of the supra-glottis—that region of the larynx which lies above the vocal cords.
2 The size of the space between the vocal cords, and the function of the vocal cords.
3 The size of the space immediately below the vocal cords.
4 The presence of pulsation in the lower trachea, suggesting a vascular abnormality.
5 The presence of any pathological swelling encroaching on the airway; this could be focal in the case of a foreign body, cyst, or general in the case of acute inflammation or allergic oedema.

TREATMENT
When this examination has been completed, the surgeon carries out any treatment which is required to safeguard the patient's airway, this may include the removal of a foreign body or tumour, the aspiration of crusts or pus from the tracheo-bronchial tree or perhaps the making of a tracheostomy; in any event the child must then be returned to the ward where it can be observed closely, where its breathing can be assisted by humidification and oxygen, and where suction is available as it is required.

In many cases no special treatment is required after the immediate post-operative period of observation. If surgical treatment is called for, the larynx may be too small at the time that the diagnosis is made for a sufficiently precise surgical technique to be employed. Under these circumstances the child may have to be kept in hospital until such time as the treatment can be completed, particularly if there is any danger of sudden obstruction to the airway. If it is necessary to make a tracheostomy it will be necessary to keep the child in hospital, as only few parents can manage a tracheostomy in a young child.

It is unnecessary in a book of this kind to give a detailed account of the many fascinating conditions which may be met with, whose presence gives rise to the symptom of stridor, but it is essential to indicate what the prognosis might be, and to outline how the case should be managed.

In the past, textbooks have stated that stridor in infancy which was present at birth was not serious and that in any case it usually cleared up at the age of two years. However, this has not been confirmed by a long-term study, which shows that only rarely does stridor cease at this age. Many of these children have feeding difficulties well on into childhood, and in addition they may have two or three attacks of chest infection every year. At the time of the attack the stridor increases in severity, and the child may need oxygen and increased humidity to assist its breathing. The fact that stridor indicates a measure of respiratory obstruction cannot be stated too frequently. The management of the case must therefore be planned with this in mind.

The parents should have the position explained to them in simple language, all drama should be avoided in order not to alarm them, but they must be made to realise that if the stridor should become worse at any time, perhaps in conjunction with an upper respiratory tract infection, then the child should be taken into hospital without delay so that adequate treatment may be provided. The child must be kept under regular observation until the stridor has disappeared, and it is not unusual to have to continue supervision until the child is five or six years old. At these regular attendances, the child is weighed and the weight compared with weights for normal children of that height and age. The chest condition is checked, and the history of troubles in-between visits obtained; if the stridor persists unaccountably then it will be necessary to carry out further endoscopic examinations. Where a stridor occurs in a previously healthy child, three possible causes should be considered:

1 Acute inflammation
2 An inhaled foreign body
3 The development of an innocent tumour such as a papilloma.

The child should be admitted to hospital immediately and steps taken to reach a diagnosis by clinical examination, and by radiology if this is necessary. Oxygen and humidification are provided and the larynx is examined by direct examination. When a cause is found, the treatment appropriate to that cause is instituted, i.e. humidification, antibiotics with or without steroids in the case of inflammation. If the obstruction is severe, then it may be necessary to assist the breathing with endotracheal intubation. In the case of foreign bodies, these must be removed as soon as the diagnosis is made. Vegetable foreign bodies are particularly dangerous for if they are left in the respiratory tract, they can set up 'vegetable pneumonia' which is rapidly fatal.

Tumours such as multiple papillomata should be removed, and if they are causing severe obstruction it may be necessary to carry out a preliminary tracheostomy.

Chapter Twenty-one

Tracheotomy and Tracheostomy

DEFINITIONS

A tracheotomy is an operation to incise the trachea. A tracheostomy is the operation whereby an opening is made in the trachea.

INDICATIONS

Tracheostomy is one of the oldest operations of surgery. Until recently it was carried out only for relief of obstruction of the larynx, but in the last twenty years a tracheostomy has been used with increasing frequency in the treatment of any patient with respiratory failure. It may thus be indicated in the following circumstances.

(a) Central lesions causing depression of the respiratory centres, the commonest being:

> Cerebro-vascular accidents.
> Barbiturate overdosage.
> Head injury.

In these patients a tracheostomy may be of help both to guard the patient from inhalation of secretions, as he is unconscious, and as an adjunct to intermittent positive pressure respiration (I.P.P.R.).

(b) Lesions of the efferent nerves controlling the muscles of respiration and lesions of the neuro-muscular junction; these include tetanus, poliomyelitis, lesions of the cervical cord and myasthenia gravis. In all these conditions there is failure of the muscles of respiration and respiration may need to be assisted by I.P.P.R. If the patient has to be maintained on a respirator for more than a day or two the airway cannot be maintained by an endotracheal tube because this causes damage to the larynx over a period of days. The airway must therefore be maintained by a cuffed tracheostomy tube.

(c) Lesions of the chest wall, the most important being multiple fractures of the ribs, causing instability of the chest wall. These patients are also treated on a respirator.

(d) Lesions of the lungs themselves. A tracheostomy tube may be of help in a patient with chronic bronchitis or emphysema, both to provide access to the lower respiratory tract for suction of viscid secretions and because the use of I.P.P.R. is indicated.

(e) Major operations on the upper respiratory tract. A tracheostomy is carried out to ensure an airway during the performance of a major cancer operation of the head and neck such as resection of the lower jaw, laryngectomy, etc.

(f) Obstruction of the airway may be due to:

Laryngeal carcinoma.

Invasion of the larynx from surrounding structures such as carcinoma of the thyroid or pharynx.

Paralysis of the vocal cords.

Foreign bodies in the larynx.

Any of the causes of laryngeal stridor in a child listed on pp. 138–41.

Airway obstruction due to these causes must be rapidly relieved by a tracheostomy.

TECHNIQUE

Tracheostomy may be carried out as an emergency operation for relief of upper respiratory obstruction or may be carried out at leisure as an elective operation.

The operation is much easier to do under general anaesthetic, but in respiratory obstruction it must be done under local anaesthetic. It should also be done if at all possible in an operating theatre with good light.

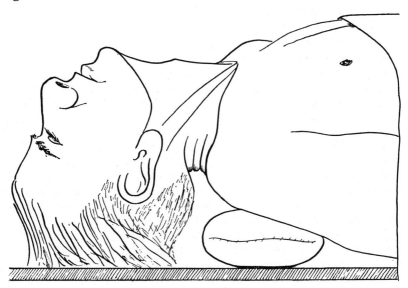

Fig. 62 Position for tracheostomy.

The patient's neck must be extended so that the trachea comes to lie immediately beneath the skin. To achieve this, the patient's shoulders should be supported by a sand-bag, although in a patient with respira-

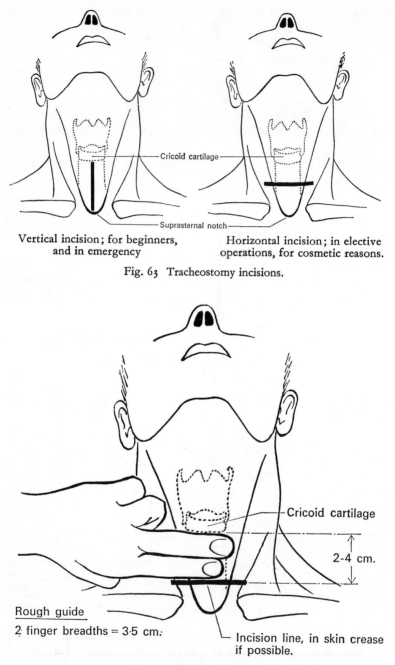

Vertical incision; for beginners, and in emergency

Horizontal incision; in elective operations, for cosmetic reasons.

Cricoid cartilage

Suprasternal notch

Fig. 63 Tracheostomy incisions.

Cricoid cartilage

2-4 cm.

Rough guide

2 finger breadths = 3·5 cm.

Incision line, in skin crease if possible.

Fig. 64 Horizontal incision for tracheostomy.

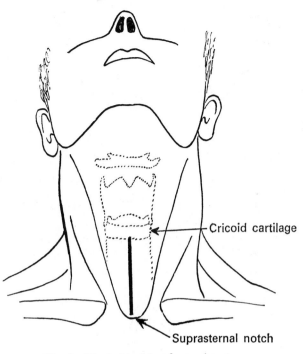

Fig. 65 Vertical incision for tracheostomy.

tory obstruction, his difficulties are increased by laying him down and extending his neck and it may not be possible to achieve this.

The skin incision for tracheotomy may be either horizontal or vertical. The horizontal incision leaves a better scar, but the operation is more difficult when carried out through this incision. If the operation is being done for the first time, particularly in an emergency, a vertical incision should be used. The incision must be strictly in the midline and extend from the level of the cricoid cartilage to the supra-sternal notch—avoid 'keyhole surgery'.

Dissection is then carried on strictly in the midline to separate the strap muscles until the trachea can be felt. The opening into the trachea must not be made in the first or second tracheal ring because of the danger of subsequent collapse of the cricoid cartilage. It is, therefore, made about the fourth tracheal ring in front of which lies the thyroid isthmus. This is divided between clamps and the divided ends of the isthmus transfixed.

If there is enough time available it is better to anaesthetise the inside of the trachea by injecting one to two millilitres of topical anaesthetic directly into the trachea.

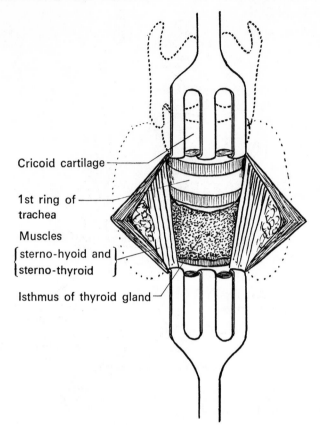

Cricoid cartilage

1st ring of
trachea

Muscles
{sterno-hyoid and}
{sterno-thyroid}

Isthmus of thyroid gland

Fig. 66 Tracheostomy. Approach to trachea.

The next step is to open the trachea. In an emergency and in a conscious patient the trachea is mobile. It is of great help to steady the
trachea by a blunt hook placed beneath the cricoid cartilage and pulled
gently but firmly towards the patient's chin.

The trachea is then opened, but before doing so all bleeding must be
controlled. In an emergency the easiest thing to do is to make a vertical
incision, through the third and fourth or fourth and fifth tracheal rings.
If there is no urgency a hole can be cut in the trachea, or a flap can be
cut, base downwards, the flap turned out and sutured to the skin.

The latter method has the advantage of ensuring that the tracheostomy is held permanently open and makes replacement of the tube
easy but it may produce granulations of the tracheal wall, leading to
scarring and stenosis. The beginner is best advised to use a vertical
slit.

The incision in the trachea must then be held open while the tube is
inserted. The easiest way of doing this is to retract both sides of the

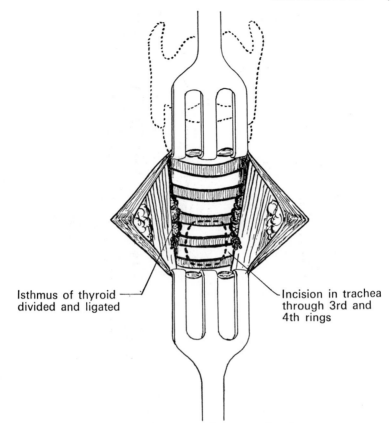

Isthmus of thyroid divided and ligated

Incision in trachea through 3rd and 4th rings

Fig. 67 Tracheostomy. Exposure of trachea.

tracheal incision with small retractors. There is also a dilator (Trousseau's) designed for this purpose but it is cumbersome for a beginner because its action is opposite to that of most forceps, i.e. the handles must be brought together to separate the points.

The tracheostomy tube is then introduced and tied in with tapes. The trachea is sucked out at this stage and the patient is then returned to the ward.

Excessive bleeding may occur during the operation due to venous congestion as a result of respiratory obstruction and therefore ceases as soon as the airway has been re-established.

In a child the innominate vessels may pass across the trachea higher than usual. It is therefore safer to open the trachea from below upwards.

AFTER-CARE
As a tracheostomy is now performed for a wide range of conditions

most junior hospital staff will need to look after one or several patients who have had this operation: success of the management of this procedure depends to a great extent on the skill of the nursing and junior medical staff.

(a) *Humidification*

The trachea and bronchi are lined by ciliated epithelium covered by a mucous blanket which is easily damaged, particularly by a blast of cold dry air, which dries the mucous blanket and paralyses the underlying cilia. The nose warms and humidifies the inspired air to prevent this. The air inspired through a tracheostomy must therefore be humidified; if it is not, crusting of secretions occurs.

Humidification may be provided either in the form of steam or 'cold steam'.

(i) Steam from a kettle is an old-fashioned method but is still satisfactory.

(ii) 'Cold steam', which is cold water converted to droplets by atomisation, is now often used. Such a humidifier can either be used in a tent or the humidified air can be supplied to the patient by a tube delivering the humidified air to the entrance to the trachea tube.

(b) *Suction*

Despite adequate humidification, secretions build up in the tracheobronchial tree and because the patient has been deprived of his own cough reflex his trachea must be sucked out through the tube. This must be carried out at frequent intervals in the first few days whenever the characteristic rattle of secretions is heard. Infection can easily be introduced into the trachea during aspiration and the following points should therefore be meticulously observed:

(i) Everybody in the region of a patient with a tracheostomy should wear a face mask; this includes senior medical staff.

(ii) The person carrying out aspiration of a tracheostomy must carry out a surgical scrub of his hands first.

(iii) Sterile disposable catheters must be used and they must not be allowed to come into contact with any surrounding articles before they are introduced into the trachea.

(iv) The aspirating catheter should be introduced with the suction turned off. If the catheter is inserted when the suction is turned on, it merely adheres to the wall of the upper trachea. When the sucker has been introduced to its limit, suction is turned on and the sucker withdrawn.

(v) Both major bronchi must be aspirated. The right main bronchus is wider and straighter than the left and the carina lies to the left of the midline so that there is a tendency to suck out the right main bronchus only. To overcome this, the patient can be tipped on to both sides or a Pinkerton catheter, which is bent at the end, can be used to ensure that both major bronchi are being aspirated.

(c) *Toilet*

Despite proper suction the tube eventually becomes blocked by secretions and must be cleaned. How this is done depends on the type of tube used.

Tracheostomy tubes may be divided into two types, those made of metal and those made of rubber or polythene. Each of these has advantages and disadvantages. All metal tubes, whatever their pattern, consist of three parts: an inner tube, an outer tube and an introducer. The inner tube is always slightly longer than the outer tube so that it

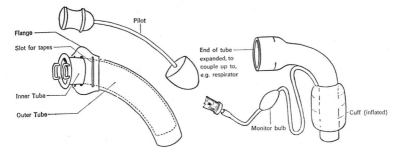

Fig. 68 Types of tracheostomy tubes. (Left) Standard metal (silver) type. (Right) Cuffed type (rubber or 'Portex').

juts out further into the trachea and crusts tend to collect on it rather than on the outer tube. The inner tube can be removed, bringing the crusts with it, leaving the outer tube to maintain the airway while the inner tube is cleaned and replaced. This is done twice a day. The ease with which the inner tube can be cleaned is the great advantage of metal tubes; their disadvantage is that they do not have an inflatable cuff.

Although the inner tube is cleaned frequently the outer tube becomes crusted eventually and should also be taken out and cleaned every few days. But the outer tube should not be taken out in the first two days if the larynx is obstructed, particularly in a child. On the first day the track is not fully established and the hole may disappear if the entire tube is taken out, so that it cannot be put back.

Tracheostomy tubes made of rubber or polythene almost all have an inflatable cuff. This is a great advantage in the patient whose breathing is being assisted by a respirator (I.P.P.R.) which requires an air tight connection of the trachea to the machine. A cuffed tube also has the advantage of preventing inhalation of food and secretions; its main disadvantage is that there is only one tube so that it must all be removed for cleaning. Also, to prevent crusting in these tubes, very careful and thorough suction is needed.

(d) *Deflation of cuff*

Although an inflatable cuff is a great advantage, the cuff itself can cause considerable damage. When fully inflated the pressure in it is 120–150 mm Hg and thus may be higher than the systolic blood pressure, causing ischaemic necrosis of the adjacent tracheal wall resulting in stenosis. Thus the cuff must be deflated for at least five minutes in every hour and must be left permanently deflated as soon as possible.

(e) *Spare tube*

A spare tube should always be left at the bedside along with a forceps and introducer so that the airway can be re-established if the tube comes out.

(f) *Feeding*

Most patients with a tracheostomy will be unable to eat because of the condition for which the operation has been done, so that tube feeding will be necessary.

An adequate intake should be given, the easiest way of doing this being to liquidise a normal diet and pour it down the tube. To make sure that the patient is being properly fed he should be weighed every few days and a strict fluid balance chart kept.

(g) *Speech*

The patient with a tracheostomy obviously cannot speak. He must therefore have a bell to attract attention in cases of emergency and will need pencil and paper. There is also available a set of plastic discs strung on a chain each bearing a useful word such as 'Bed-pan', 'Spectacles', etc.

COMPLICATIONS

(a) *Apnoea*

If a patient has had respiratory obstruction for several weeks, carbon dioxide accumulates in the alveoli and the respiratory centre accommodates to an increased concentration of carbon dioxide in the blood. When the trachea is opened carbon dioxide is rapidly washed out, the concentration in the blood falls and breathing may stop. It can be re-started either by artificial respiration or by giving the patient 5 % carbon dioxide in air to breathe.

(b) *Bleeding*

Secondary haemorrhage may occur because of infection round the tracheostomy site and can be controlled by antibiotics.

Occasionally a metal tube, if it is incorrectly angled, erodes the anterior wall of the trachea and ruptures the innominate artery. This accident is inevitably and immediately fatal. It should be suspected to be imminent if there is a small bleed of fresh blood from within the trachea a few days after tracheostomy. The disaster might then be averted by changing to a portex or rubber tube.

(c) *Damage to the oesophagus*
The party wall between the oesophagus and trachea is membranous. If the trachea is incised during inspiration, the party wall may at that time be drawn forward and damaged. This tends to happen only in an urgent tracheostomy.

(d) *Damage to the cricoid cartilage*
If the tracheostomy is established in the first or second tracheal rings, chondritis of the cricoid cartilage may occur. The cartilage collapses, and the patient's airway is then permanently useless. This accident should be avoided by placing the tracheostomy below the second tracheal ring.

(e) *Surgical emphysema of the neck and chest*
If the skin is stitched tightly round a tracheostomy, air can get out around the hole in the trachea but cannot get out through the skin. It therefore passes into the tissues. Thus the skin must not be tightly sutured. If surgical emphysema occurs, the stitches should be released.

(f) *Pneumothorax*
A pneumothorax occurs fairly often after an urgent tracheostomy. It is usually due to rupture of a bulla caused by increased respiratory efforts during obstruction. A chest X-ray should always be taken after a tracheotomy has been done.

(g) *Pressure necrosis*
Ischaemic necrosis of the trachea causing a stenotic ring may occur after the use of a cuffed tube if the cuff is inflated for too long.

STRIDOR AFTER TRACHEOSTOMY
Stridor in a patient with a tracheostomy may be caused by the tube being displaced to lie in the soft tissues of the neck or by the tube being blocked by secretions. If stridor occurs the tube should, therefore, be checked to see that it is in the right place and that it is clean.

DECANNULATION
Many tracheostomies are carried out for temporary, reversible condi-

tions. The tracheostomy must be closed as soon as possible because the patient is in constant danger of infection while it is in place.

Decannulation can be achieved by progressive corking of the tube or by substituting smaller and smaller tubes, but in many cases it can be removed without further ado. The tube should be completely blocked for twenty-four hours before removing it. If the patient can sleep, eat and walk without stridor it is then safe to remove the tube. Another useful practical guide is the absence of stridor. The patient is asked to take a deep breath with his mouth open. If no stridor is present the tube can safely be removed.

Decannulation in infants may be difficult. There are several reasons why this may be. Infection or necrosis of tracheal cartilage inevitably causes slight narrowing of the trachea. In the large trachea of an adult this is of no importance, but it causes a relatively large loss of lumen in the infant's narrow trachea. Part of the problem may also be psychological because the child has become used to breathing through his tracheostomy and cannot readjust to normal breathing.

Appendix 1

Examples of Audiograms

For a description of Audiometry see p. 7.
Conductive deafness (see p. 38)

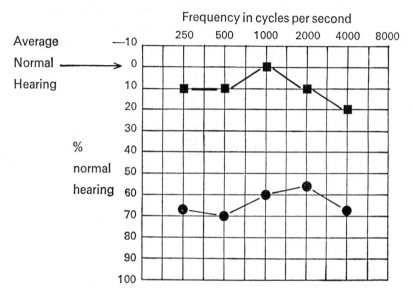

Sensory-neural deafness (see p. 39)

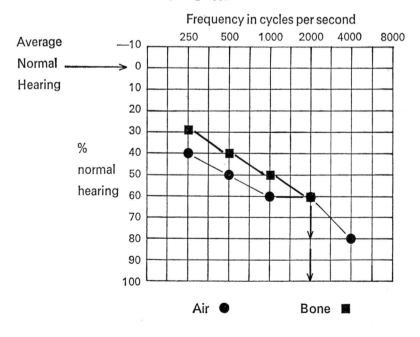

Index

ISBN 0 340 18890 1   Paperback

First printed 1971
Reprinted 1972
Second edition 1974
Tenth impression 1986

Printed and bound in Great Britain
for Hodder and Stoughton Educational,
a division of Hodder and Stoughton Ltd,
Mill Road, Dunton Green, Sevenoaks, Kent,
by Richard Clay (The Chaucer Press), Ltd., Bungay, Suffolk